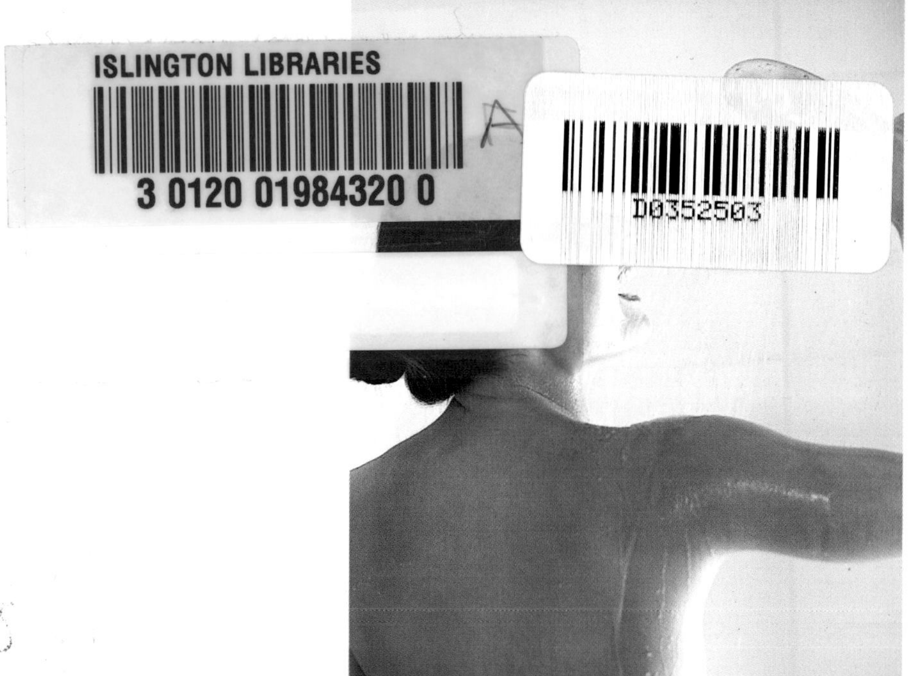

wake-up workout

Jacqueline Lysycia

wake-up workout

10 MINUTES A DAY TO A BETTER BODY

hamlyn

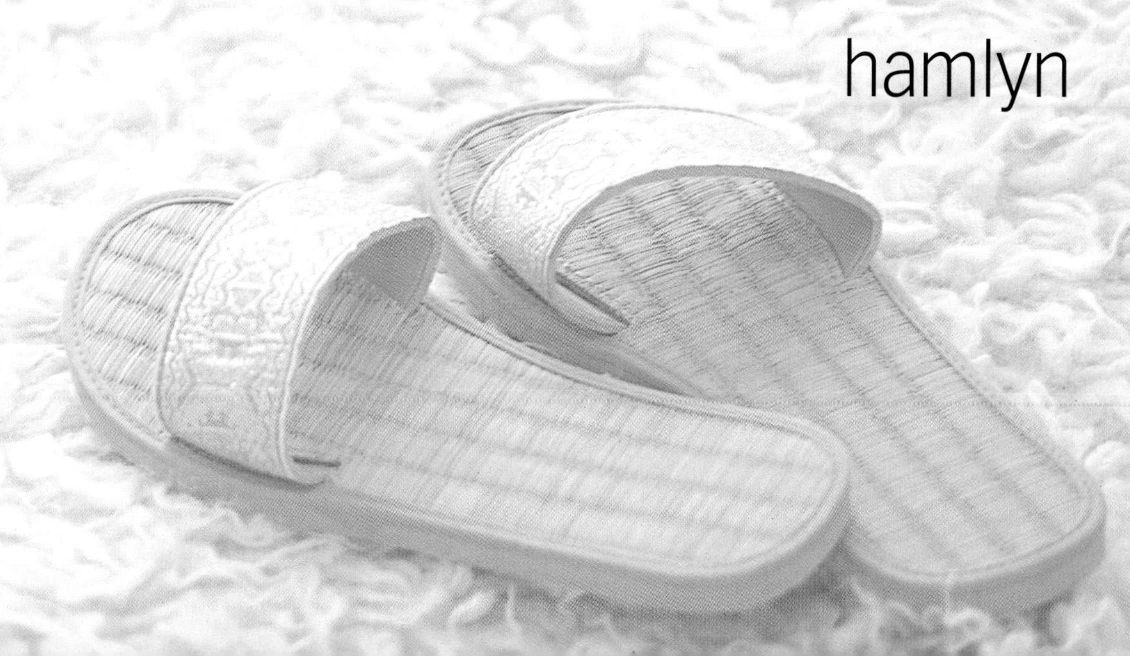

First published in Great Britain in 2005 by
Hamlyn, a division of Octopus Publishing Group Ltd
2–4 Heron Quays, London E14 4JP

Distributed in the United States and Canada by
Sterling Publishing Co., Inc.
387 Park Avenue South, New York, NY
10016–8810

ISBN 0 600 61193 0
EAN 9780600611936

A CIP catalogue record for this book is available from the British Library

Printed and bound in Spain

10 9 8 7 6 5 4 3 2 1

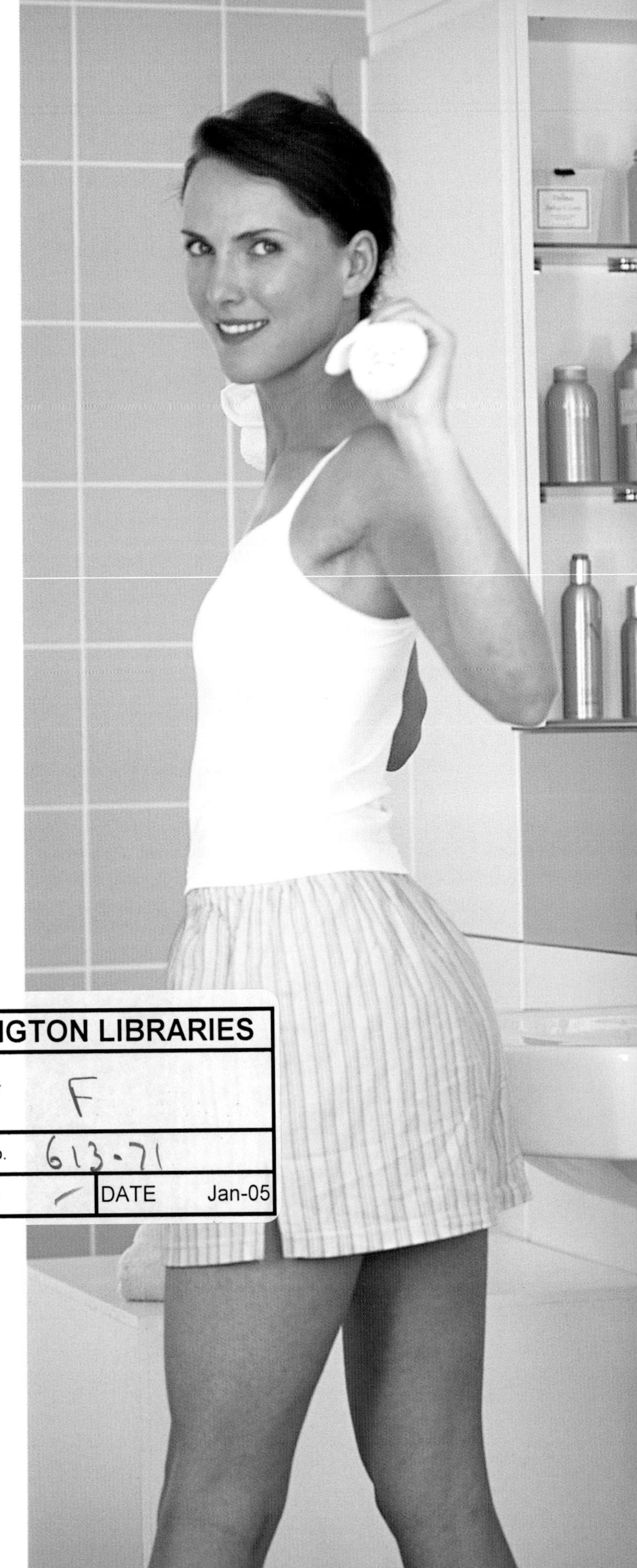

Note

It is advisable to check with your physici[...] embarking on any exercise programme. A physician should be consulted on all matters relating to health and any symptoms which may require diagnosis or medical attention. While the advice and information in this book is believed to be accurate and the instructions given have been devised to avoid strain, neither the author nor the publisher can accept any legal responsibility for any injury sustained while following the exercises.

contents

introduction

Welcome to this carefully devised programme of wake-up workouts, a series of 10-minute exercise routines guaranteed to shape the new you! Whether you are the kind of person who bounds out of bed every morning or someone who has to drag themself out from under the duvet, these mini workouts will help you kick-start your day. You don't have to get dressed and you certainly won't need trainers, which is what makes the programme so easy to use.

10-minute sessions

Exercising regularly is the single most important thing you can do to promote physical and mental fitness and keep stress at bay. Exercise can help cut your risk of heart attacks and help prevent osteoporosis. It makes you sleep better, boosts your energy levels, raises your self-esteem and ensures you look and feel great. So why do most of us do so little?

Lack of time is one of the main reasons, but what if you could get all the benefits of exercise in just 10 minutes a day? In the past, experts recommended that adults undertake more than 30 continuous 'sweaty' minutes of aerobic activity at least three times per week to improve their cardiovascular fitness and body fat index. But traditional research has been superseded by modern guidelines. The American College of Sports Medicine (ACSM) now recommends that we accumulate 30–60 minutes of moderately intense physical activity most days of the week – and you don't have to do it all in one go, which is great news for the time-impoverished.

Indeed, a study by the American College of Nutrition (2001) has shown that several smaller bouts of exercise in a day are just as beneficial as one longer workout with regard to aerobic fitness and weight loss. The wake-up workout programme with its 10-minute exercise sessions is therefore ideal, not only if you have little time (or enthusiasm) to spare but also if you are currently not used to exercising.

Consistency is the key to success in any exercise programme. You will soon see a difference in your energy and fitness levels with wake-up workouts, even more so once you can establish a routine involving a 10-minute workout every morning and another one or two 10-minute sessions later in the day.

Why the wake-up workout?

The wake-up workout programme is based around the theory of exercising first thing to kick-start your metabolism. The workouts are therefore best performed in the morning but can be done at other times of the day.

Make a habit of getting to bed 10 minutes earlier so you can find time in the morning to exercise without losing any sleep at all. You will soon discover how easy it is to wake up and exercise, and quickly see the results – you'll feel stronger, more toned and less stressed – which provide even more motivation to work out every morning. What's more, you have seven different types of wake-up exercise to choose from every day so you won't get bored.

CALORIE BURNING

The number of calories you burn when exercising depends greatly on your metabolism, weight and exercise history, but as a rough guideline you can expect to burn the following calories while doing the workouts in this book:

Warm-ups	150–200
Cool-downs	80–120
Rise and shine	100–200
Yoga	150–250
Cardio workout	150–250
Body sculpting	200–350
Pilates	150–250
Abdominal activators	150–250

These figures are based upon approximate calculations of 10 minutes carrying out the above activities in association with the ACSM 2004 guidelines for heart rate, flexibility and strength training.

‘With a 10-minute wake-up workout you can boost your metabolism for the rest of the day, thus burning more calories than you would if you simply rolled out of bed, via the toaster and coffee maker on the way to work’

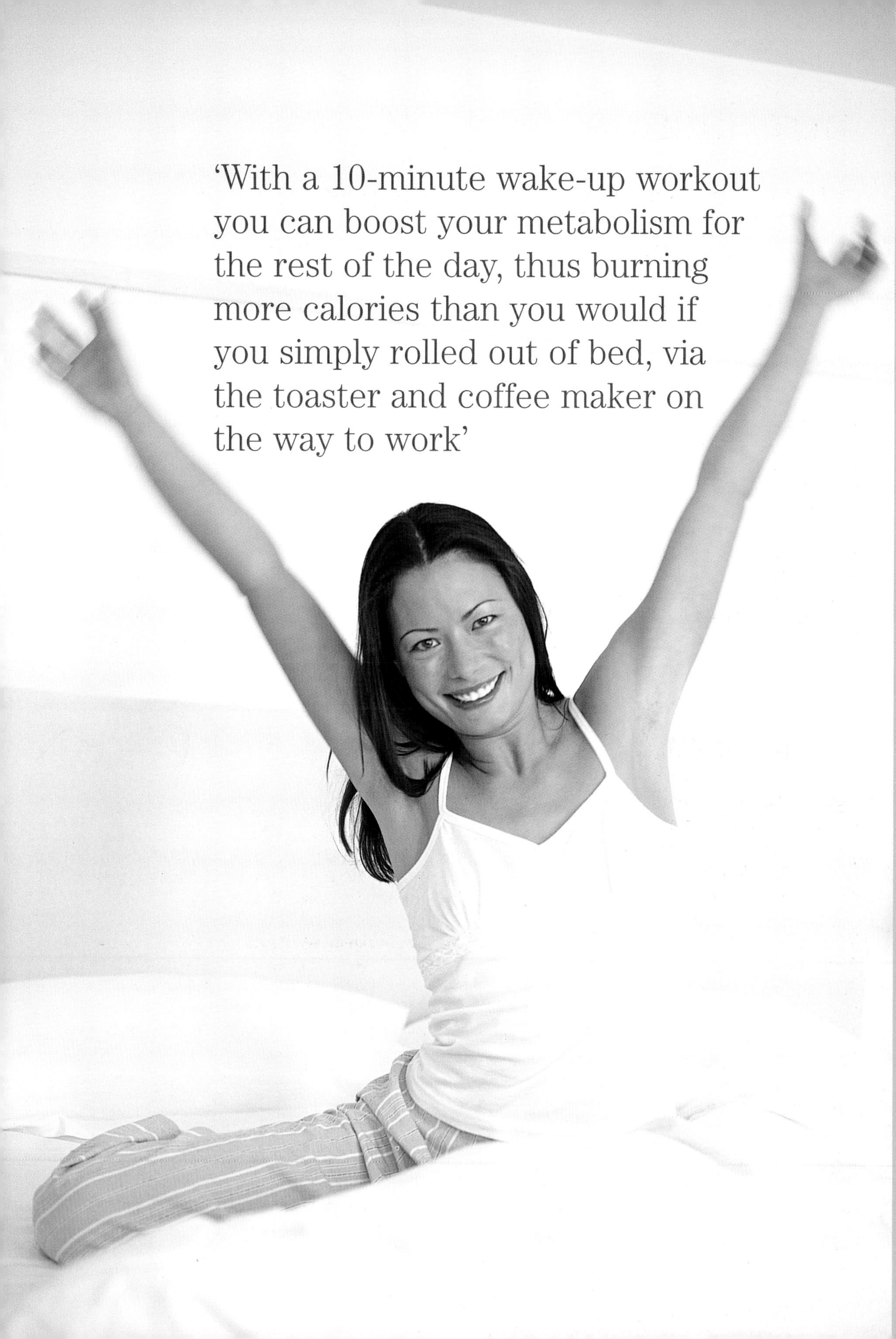

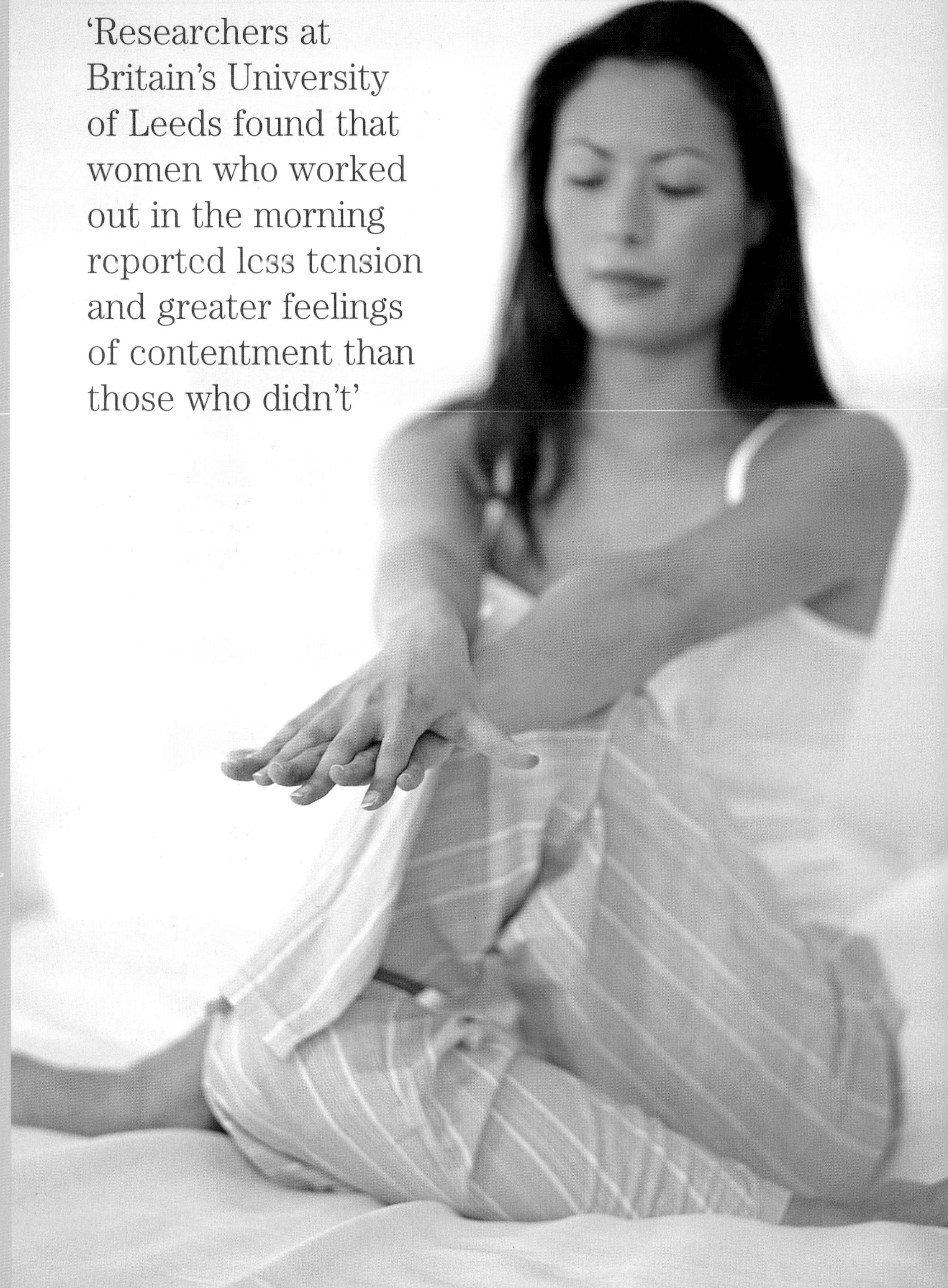

'Researchers at Britain's University of Leeds found that women who worked out in the morning reported less tension and greater feelings of contentment than those who didn't'

WHY EXERCISE IN THE MORNING?

- It boosts the metabolism
- Feel-good endorphins are released earlier in the day
- You start the day taking care of yourself
- It's an easy-to-remember, habit-forming schedule
- You achieve something soon after waking
- There are fewer distractions

Benefits of morning exercise

You probably already know how great you feel after doing your routine chores early in the day. You can relax knowing that all the important things have been covered. It's the same with morning exercise – you can be pleased with what you have achieved. More importantly, however, according to the latest research, physiologically there are more benefits to be had from exercising in the morning than at any other time of the day.

When you first wake your metabolism is sluggish because it has slowed down while you were sleeping. When you exercise, your metabolism increases. Thus, exercising in the morning enhances your metabolism when it is naturally at its lowest and it will start burning calories/fat sooner and therefore for longer during the day. A raised metabolism also increases blood supply to the brain, thereby improving your mental acuity for hours.

Exercising sends a signal to the pituitary gland in your brain to release endorphins, your body's natural feel-good drug. Exercise in the morning delivers these endorphins to your bloodstream early on, setting you up for the rest of the day.

Further advantages include the fact that after morning exercise you will feel good throughout the day because you spent some time on yourself. Whether your goal is weight loss, improved strength, relief from back pain or simply to feel better, you begin your day with a feeling of accomplishment. You are also more likely to be consistent with morning exercise as research has shown that it is easier to form habits at this time of the day (Journal of Gerentology, 1997). Most people know where they will be first thing in the morning and can make exercise a part of their getting-up routine. Lastly, there are fewer distractions first thing. Later in the day, things that demand your time will crop up and make it harder to find the time to exercise.

Who are the workouts for?

Wake-up workouts are ideal for anyone who finds it difficult to fit exercise into their regular lifestyle. They are especially beneficial for women aged 30–70. Whether you are old or young, fat or thin, tired or energetic, this programme of workouts will help you reach your exercise goals in just 10 minutes per day. There is something for everyone as the workouts offered are so varied, and the simple and easy-to-use steps will get you going instantly.

All of the sections are suited to all body types and fitness levels – let your body decide what it wants to do. The Pilates section (see pages 88–99) includes movements for those who suffer with back pain or who need to strengthen the core muscles of their abdomen and spine. The yoga section (see pages 52–67) offers stress relief and opening movements for the joints and muscles.

HEED YOUR BODY

Always consult a physician before embarking on any new exercise programme or diet plan.

Do not exercise if you:

- Have been taking painkillers as these mask any health warning signs
- Feel unwell
- Have been drinking alcohol
- Are in pain from an injury. Always consult your physician first, as rest may be needed

the essentials

Take time to read the chapters and practise the exercises individually before attempting a whole workout as it is simply not advisable to be practising 'how to' movements in the morning when you don't have much spare time.

Workouts for everyone

Some people are natural early risers, some are reluctant early risers and others are always groggy on rising. There will also be days when your routine is upset and you may feel different from usual. There are therefore seven different wake-up workouts to choose from, to suit your exercise requirements, your nature or your mood on waking (see right):

- Warm-ups and cool-downs (these are optional and are workouts in themselves) (pages 14–29)
- Rise and shine (pages 30–51)
- Wake up with yoga (pages 52–67)
- Cardio workout (pages 68–77)
- Body sculpting (pages 78–87)
- Pilates (pages 88–99)
- Abdominal activators (pages 100–109)

Starting out

Start with the warm-ups and cool-downs (see pages 14–29) as 10-minute routines in themselves. Then, when you have managed to get these down to a matter of just minutes, try the rise and shine workout (see pages 30–51). When you can competently do all the warm-ups and cool-downs and the rise and shine bedroom and bathroom routines you are ready to practise any of the other wake-up workouts. Try to stick to your 10 minutes and leave out what you don't have time for. The important thing is to get into a routine of rolling out of bed and into gentle activity. Have your breakfast after your workout (see page 70–71).

Moving on

When you are familiar with all the exercises, simply decide on waking which workout you want to undertake. Assess the realistic time you have available and choose the level you want to work at. You may want to pick some of the more fitness-orientated workouts, for example, cardio, body sculpting or abdominal exercises. Or, if you awake feeling heavy or sluggish, you could choose to stay in bed and complete the specially designed exercises without even having to get changed or put on a pair of trainers.

If you have time or want to vary your workout you can perform any of the warm-up and cool-down exercises around your chosen routine – it is up to you. Essentially, the more you move the higher your metabolism. If you are active at the beginning of your day then you will be energetic for the rest of it, too. Bear in mind that the yoga and Pilates exercises don't require a warm-up or cool-down as these movements have already been built into the routines.

Once you have worked through all the routines in the book you may like to put together a workout that combines all your favourite exercises. However, be careful not to get stuck in a rut of performing only those movements you are good at. Sometimes it is the movements you don't enjoy so much that provide the most benefit.

If you are really short of time or just want instant energy you can spritz awake or use hydrotherapy techniques to get you started (see page 32–33).

Preparation

Make sure that when you wake up you can just slide out of bed and get on with your workout. Having to clear away clutter first will be another obstacle that eats up valuable workout time. So before you go to bed ensure you have prepared your space and 'equipment' as necessary. You might need:

- A yoga mat or padded exercise mat
- A folded pillow or towel
- Loose comfortable clothing and bare feet
- A warm and light space

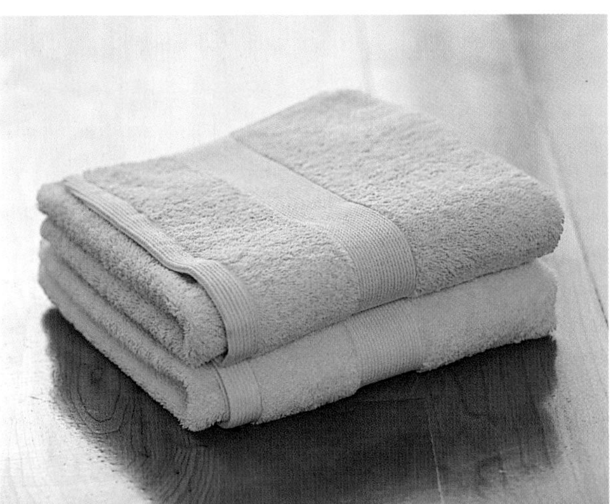

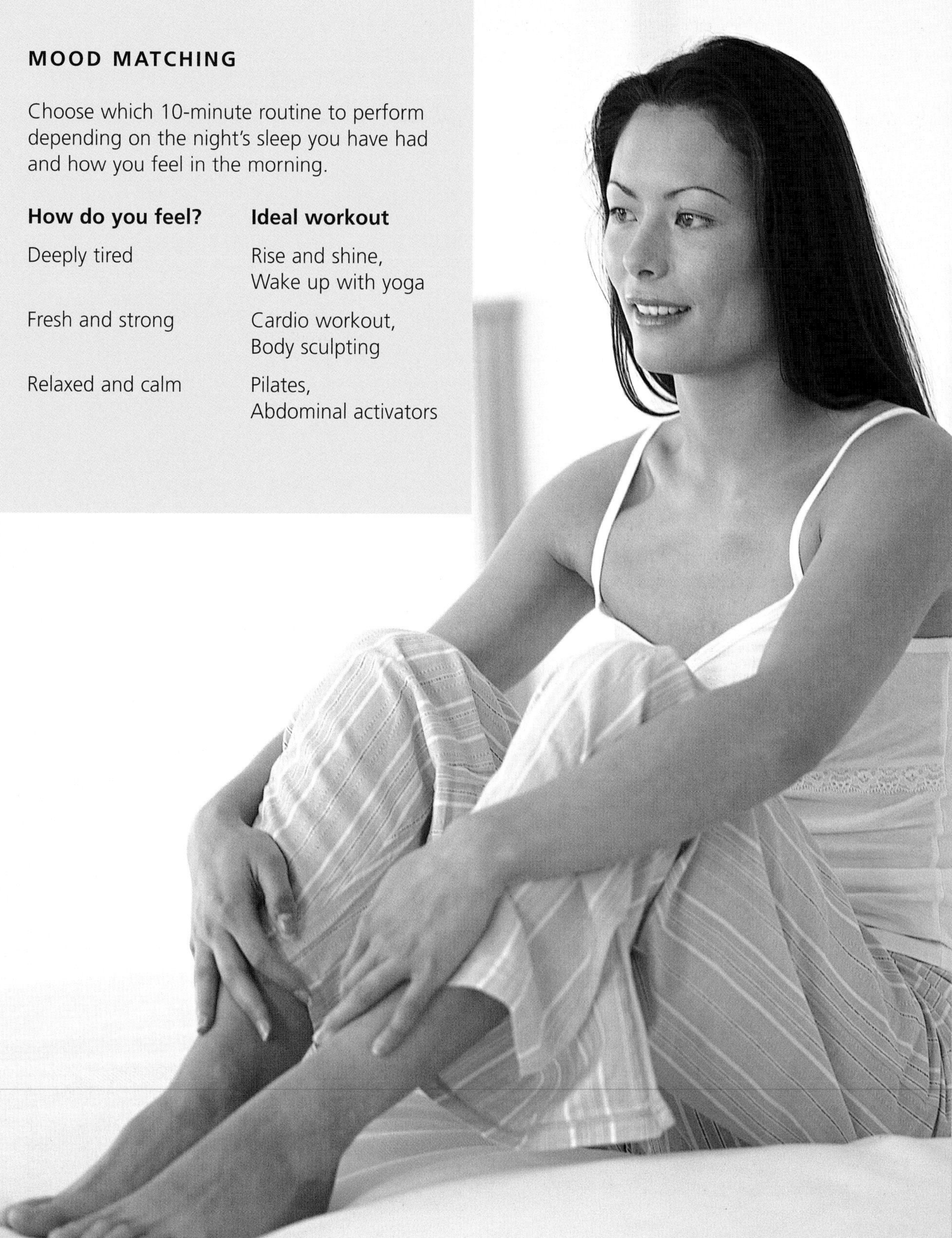

MOOD MATCHING

Choose which 10-minute routine to perform depending on the night's sleep you have had and how you feel in the morning.

How do you feel?	Ideal workout
Deeply tired	Rise and shine, Wake up with yoga
Fresh and strong	Cardio workout, Body sculpting
Relaxed and calm	Pilates, Abdominal activators

get enough sleep

A good night's sleep is essential for feeling good the following day. On average, adults function best on a regular seven or eight hours sleep a night – less and you are likely to be tired, irritable and inefficient, more and you feel woolly-headed and inert. If you wake naturally, without an alarm, feeling completely rested, then you are getting the right amount of sleep.

Stress and sleep

You might be getting less sleep than you need because of stress. Relentlessly turning things over in your mind and being unable to switch off is the classic sign. Looking after your body and taking regular physical exercise helps keep stress at bay, but you also need to make time for mental retreat.

A traditional way to calm the mind is through the ancient practice of meditation. Simple techniques such as being aware of your breathing will help your mind to become quiet. If it takes you longer than 20 minutes to drift off to sleep, refer to the 'Revitalizing breathing' on page 34. A calming bath at bedtime is also useful for inducing sleep.

'Getting into a regular sleep routine is the best way to relax and feel good'

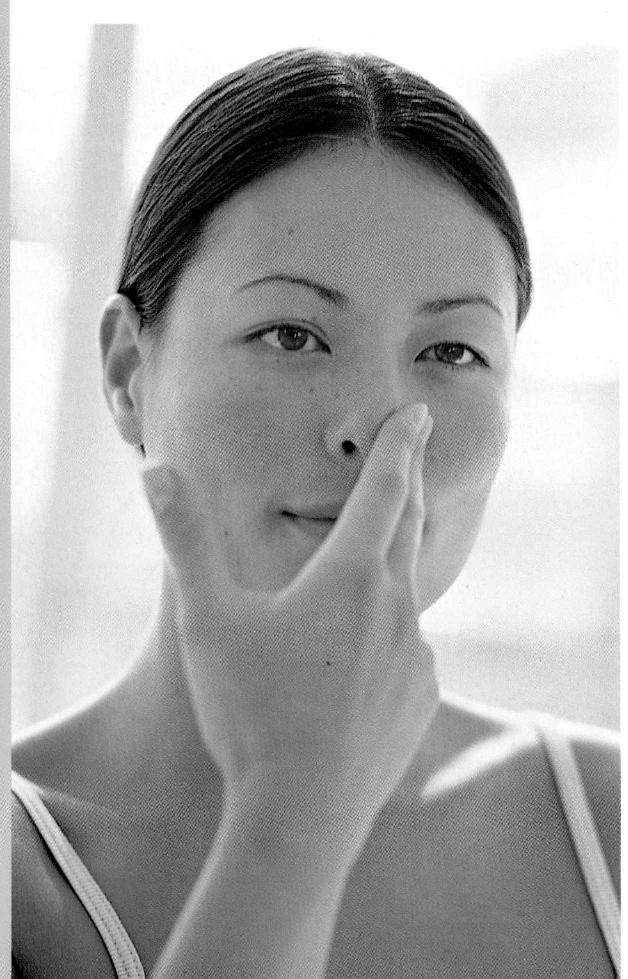

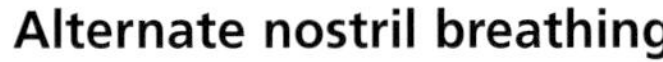

Alternate nostril breathing

This is a breathing exercise that calms the nervous system and heart rate and lowers blood pressure. It will help you to sleep and put worries away for the night where they belong.

1 Sit cross-legged on the floor or kneel with a cushion underneath your thighs.

2 Press the lip of your right nostril gently shut with your right thumb and inhale through your left nostril.

3 At the end of the inhalation, close your left nostril with the first two fingers of your right hand as you hold your breath. Remove your thumb from your right nostril and exhale.

4 Inhale through your right nostril.

5 At the end of the inhalation, remove your fingers from your left nostril and exhale.

6 Repeat this exercise slowly 10–15 times.

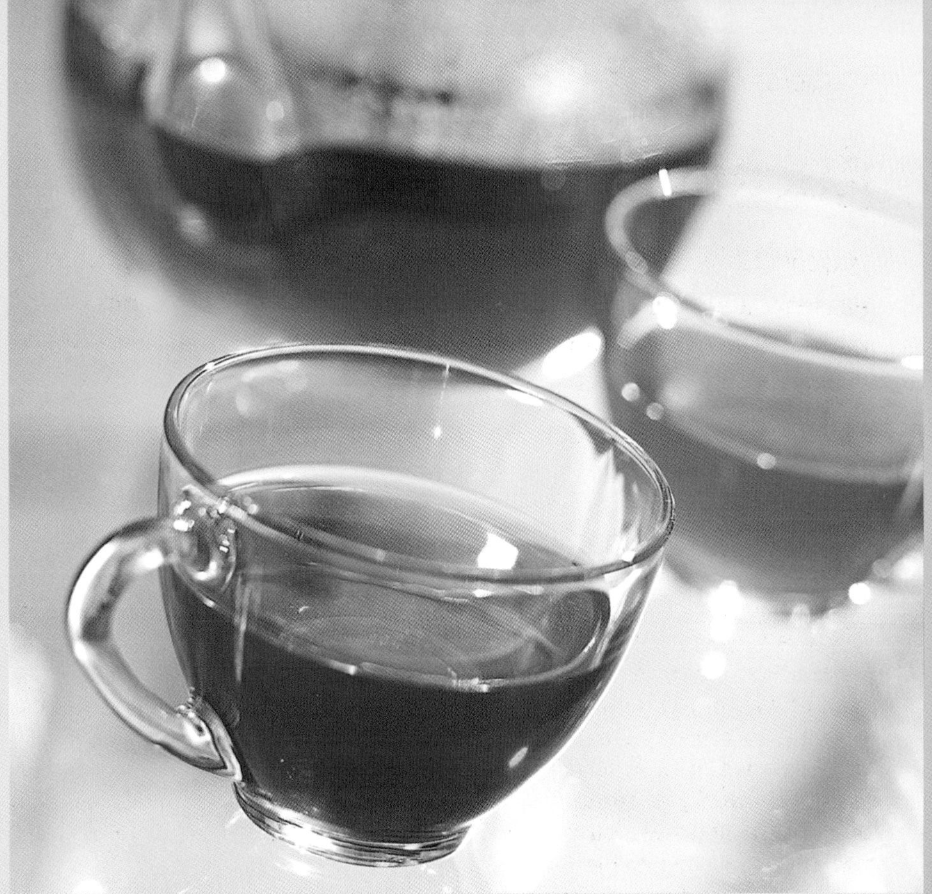

WIND DOWN GENTLY

Sleep is a great healer and stress buster, so give yourself all the help you can get.

To ensure a good night's sleep:

- Base your evening meal on good carbohydrate foods such as baked potatoes, rice and vegetables
- Have your evening meal at least two hours before bedtime
- Avoid tea, coffee, cola and even hot chocolate after 7pm. Have milky or herbal drinks instead
- Take regular exercise but not too close to bedtime
- Unwind before getting into bed to get you in the mood for sleep – read a book, have a bath or listen to some music
- Create a restful environment in your bedroom. It should be quiet and dark, and a work-, clutter- and television-free zone
- If you wake in the night and cannot get back to sleep, get up and do something relaxing such as reading. If worries keep you awake, offload them by writing them down to deal with the following day. Go back to bed when you feel sleepy

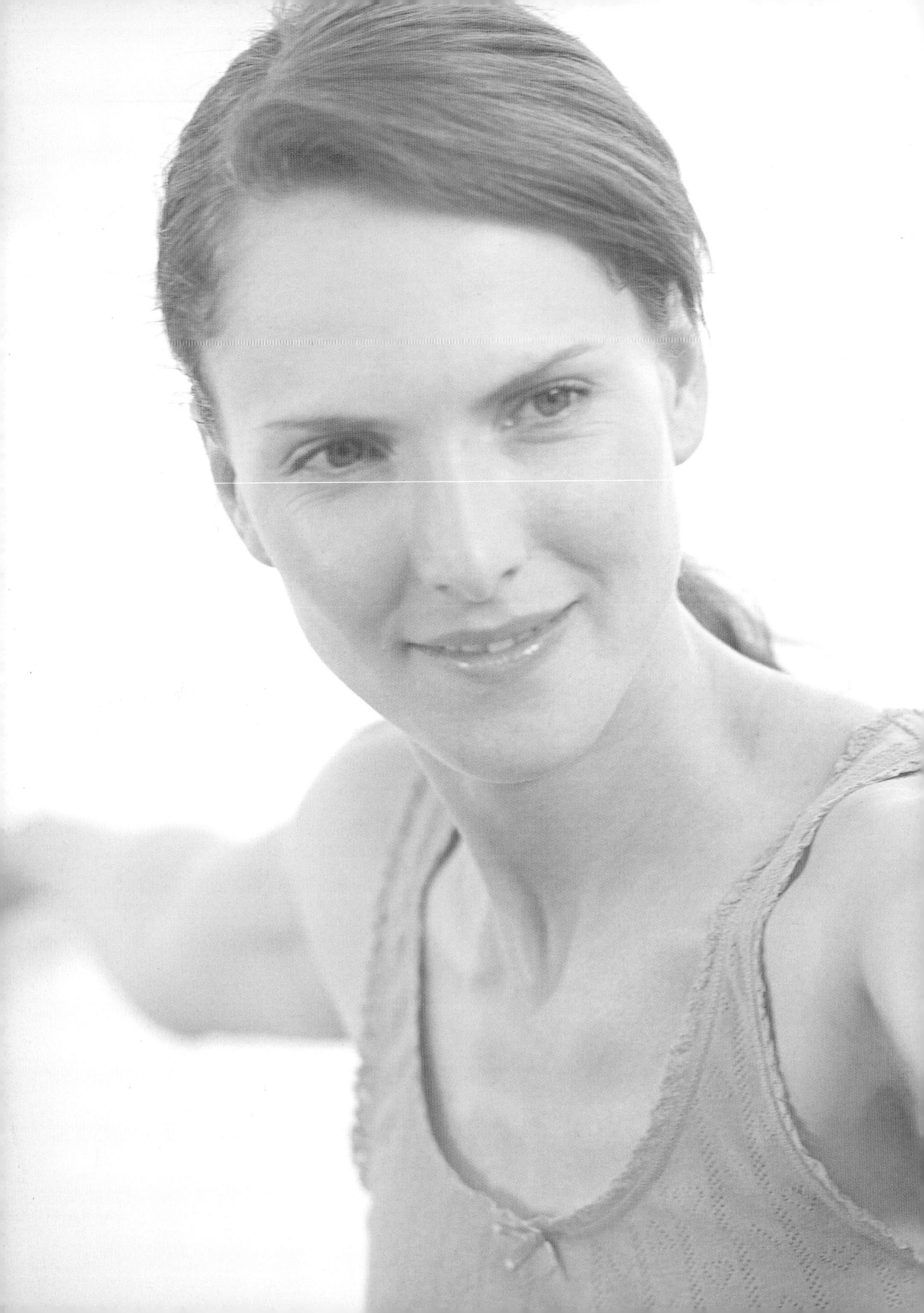

warm-ups and cool-downs

warm-ups and cool-downs

The warm-up and cool-down exercises on the following pages can be done as 10-minute workouts in themselves or you can choose any movements from this chapter to help you prepare for and/or finish another of the wake-up workouts.

Why warm up?

Your body lies dormant for seven or eight hours during your nightly sleep so your muscles and joints are a little stiff in the morning and your blood supply and circulation take a while to wake up because oxygen demand during sleep is low. Warm-up exercises are therefore advisable to gently – and safely – awaken your body before more vigorous exercising. The exercises will soften interconnective tissue before any intense movements are performed. The spine, for example, is the backbone of our whole structure and must be gently awakened. In fact, all of the 10-minute wake-up workouts only use those movements that are friendly to your body in the morning.

A warm-up routine will also prepare you mentally and help you to focus on your 10-minute workout plan more efficiently. The better you warm up and prepare, the more endorphins (your body's natural feel-good drug) will be released into your bloodstream, and the better you will feel. Your day will just keep on getting better and better!

At first you may find that the complete warm-up routine will take you 10 minutes, but as you become stronger, fitter and more familiar with the exercises it will take you only a few minutes and you can combine any or all of the movements with another of the wake-up workout routines.

WAKE-UP WORKOUT TERMINOLOGY

Abdominal hollowing This involves drawing your navel towards your spine so as to engage your abdominal muscles. You should still be able to breathe normally while holding this position.

Engage/switch on This means pulling in, or contracting, a muscle. 'Zip up/in' means the same thing and is the term widely used in Pilates.

Neutral The neutral position ensures the spine is bone loading centrally so that pressure is applied equally to the whole spine. It engages the transversus abdominis (pelvic floor muscles), which are the muscles responsible for our true functional core strength.

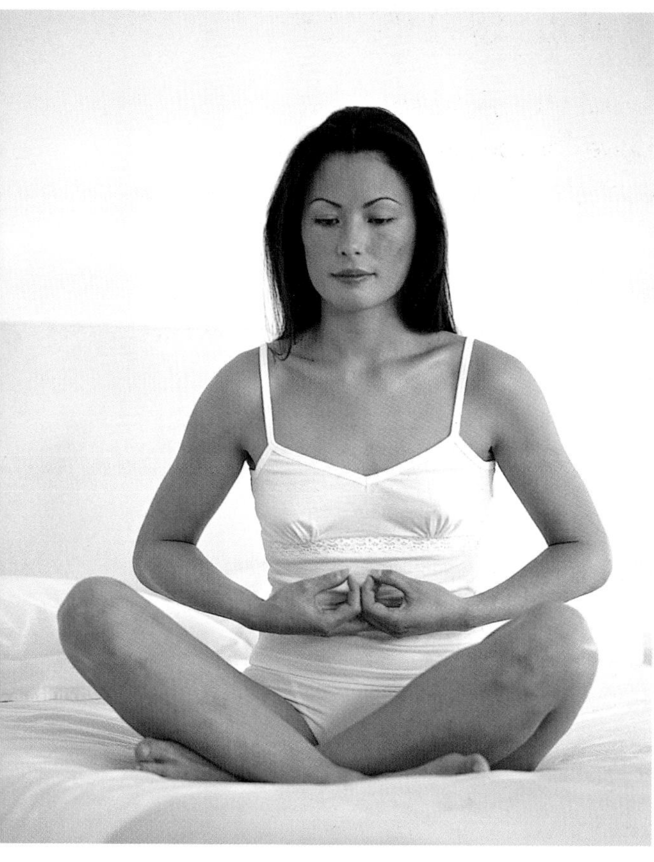

'Warm-up exercises will gently, and safely, awaken your body before more vigorous exercising'

Mental cleansing

This exercise will help you to prepare your mind for the day ahead.

1 Sit with a cushion under your sacrum (tail bone) so that your hip bones are up and forward of your pubic bone. Ensure that shinbones are rolled towards the floor. This opens the hips.

2 Take steady slow breaths and, over the course of 10 breathing cycles, gradually slow down your exhalation. Each time you breathe in, open your rib cage a bit more and feel your lungs expand. Focus on your breath only.

Why cool down?

It is advisable to perform cool-down exercises after a vigorous workout to ensure that any tension has been released from your muscles and joints. Cool-downs also help to release lactic acid, which is produced when you exercise. The lactic acid can accumulate in your muscles, particularly during a cardio workout, and if it isn't removed from your system during a cool-down session, your muscles will be left feeling stiff.

You don't have to complete the cool-down every day, but it is useful on days when you have a little more time and you may like to use it to vary your workouts. As with the warm-ups, the whole cool-down routine may take you 10 minutes to start with but will soon take you only a few minutes. You can perform the whole cool-down or just select your favourite exercises to do after another workout.

WARM-UPS AND COOL-DOWNS

Warm-ups

Cool-downs

rug ullolas

This exercise helps soften the muscles in the spine and begins to warm your trunk, legs and arms.

1 Kneel on all fours with your hands flat on the floor directly beneath your shoulders and your hips directly above your knees (the so-called box position). Spread your fingers on the floor to take your weight evenly.

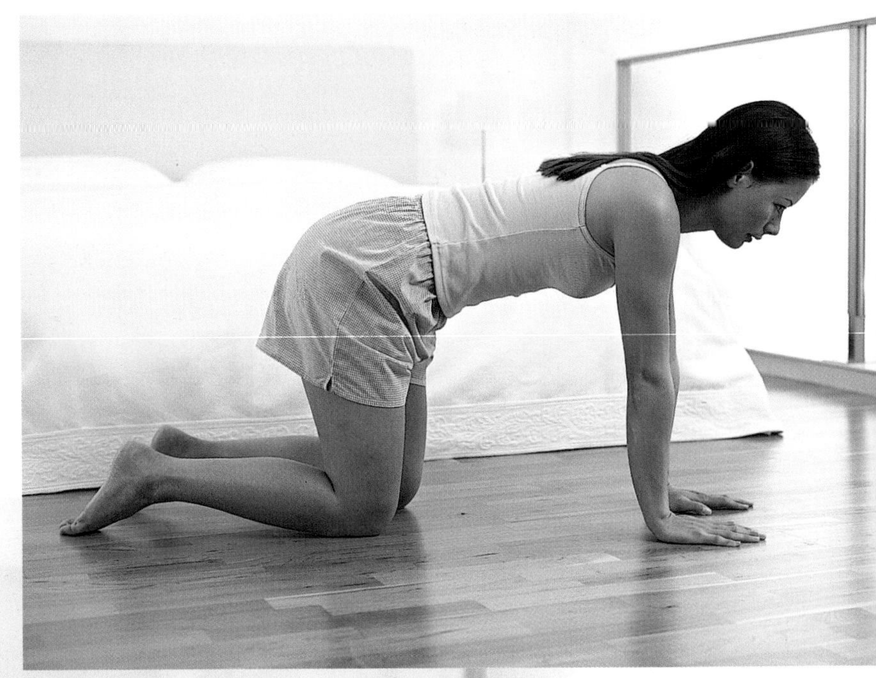

2 Take a deep breath to fill your rib cage. As you exhale, gently move your buttocks back to rest on your heels. Pull your abdomen in towards your spine as you do so and stretch your arms out in front of you on the floor.

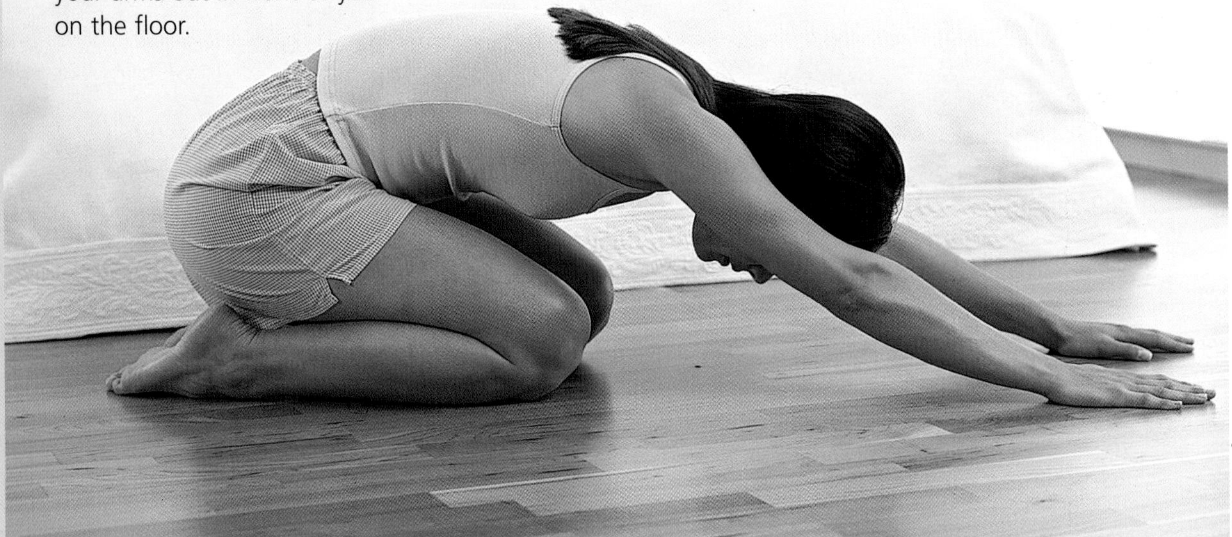

3 Inhale as you raise yourself back into the box position of Step 1.

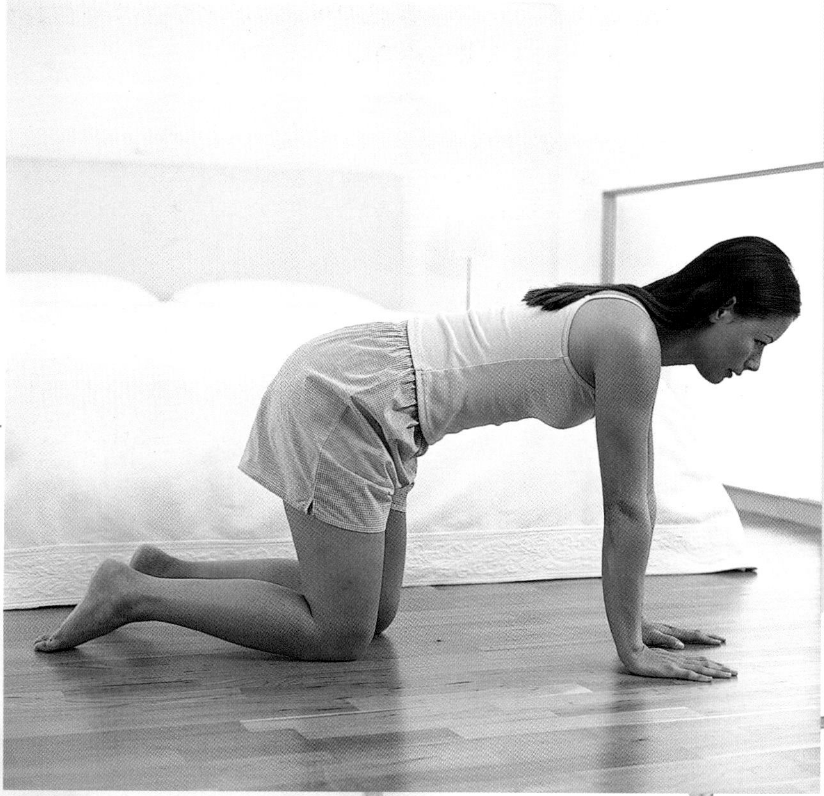

4 As you exhale bend your elbows and press your trunk down towards the floor – but don't touch it, keeping your elbows close to your body and directly above your wrists. Keep your head in line with your spine. Inhale as you push back up to the box position again. Repeat the sequence 5–10 times, keeping your breathing natural.

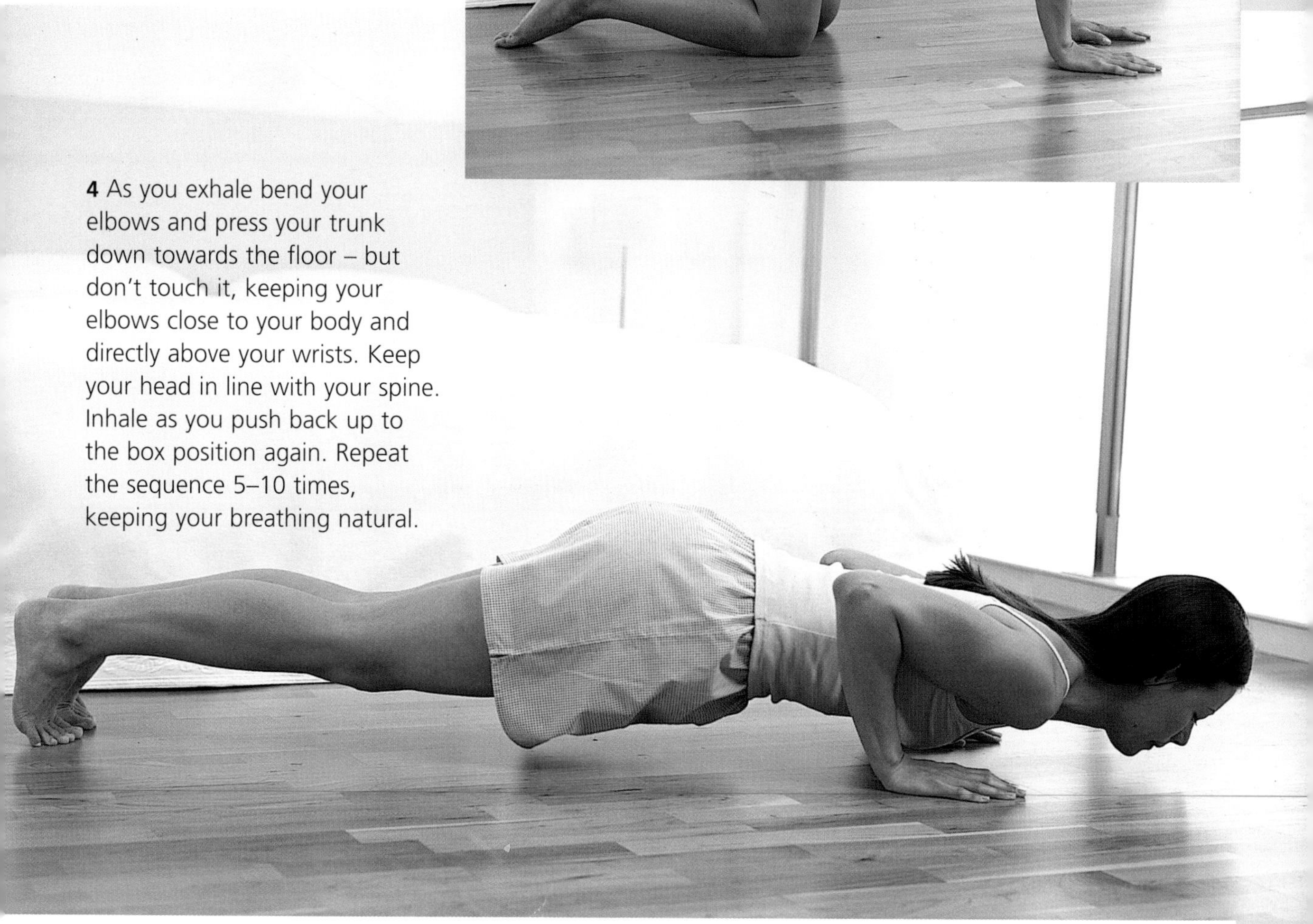

saw spine rotators

This movement increases rotation around the spine while toning your abdominals.

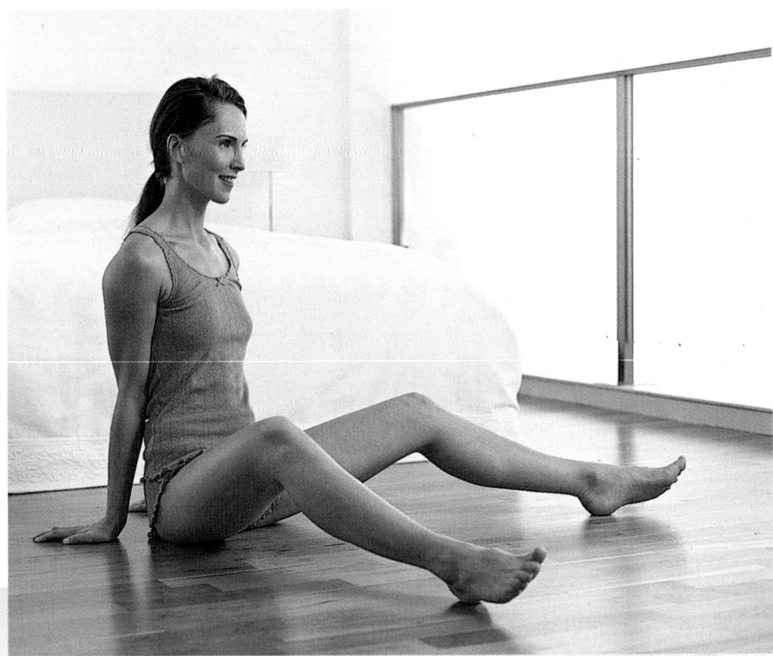

1 Sit on the floor with your legs outstretched in front of you, as far apart as is comfortable. Ensure the bones in your buttocks are grounded and press the backs of your knees towards the floor. Keep your spine erect and hollow your abdominals by pulling them in towards your spine.

2 Inhale and extend your arms out to your sides in line with your shoulders. Exhale and flatten your abdomen towards your spine.

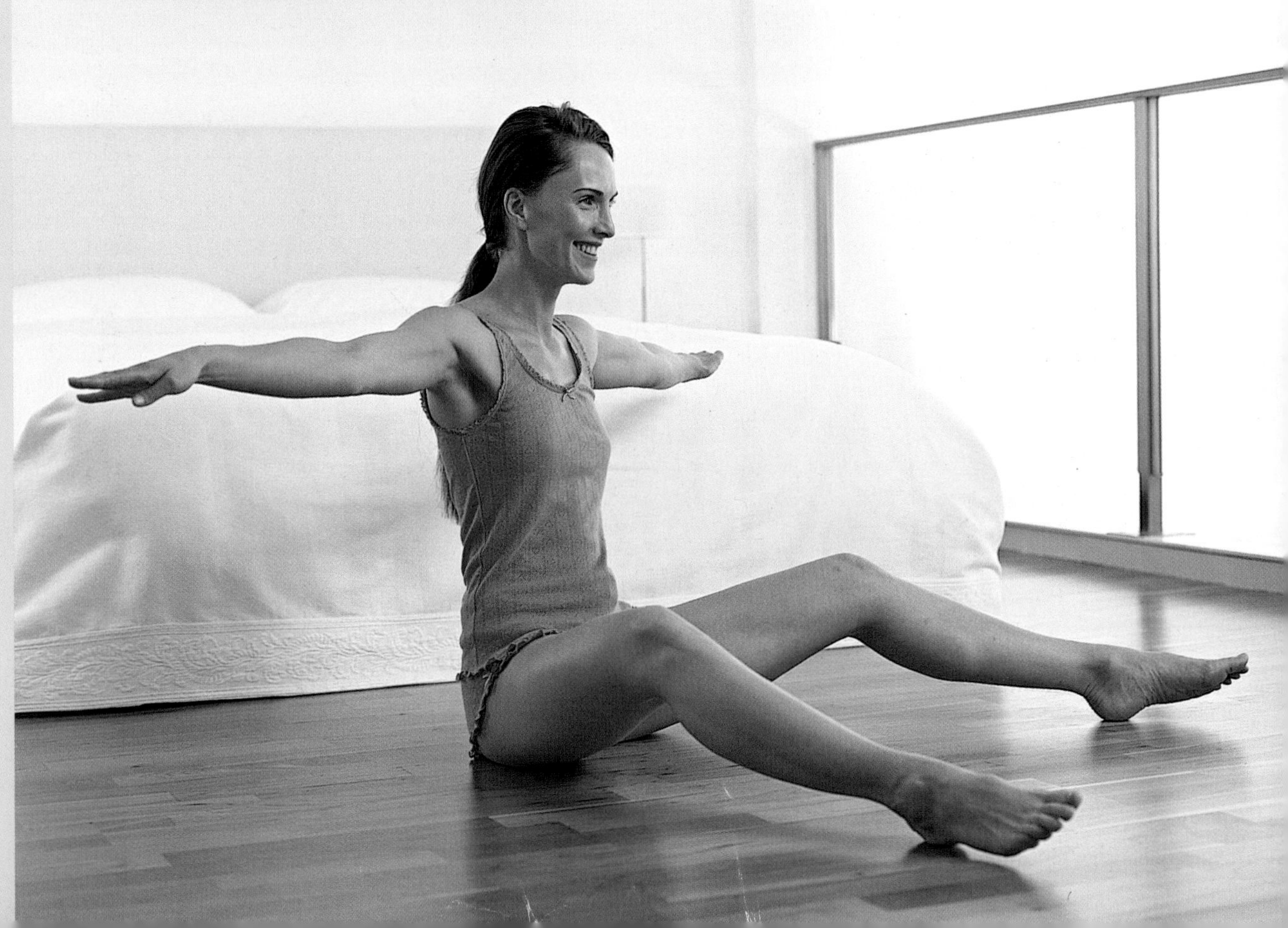

3 Inhale and rotate your trunk to one side, keeping your arms extended and your chest open. Keep your thigh muscles pulled into your thigh bones.

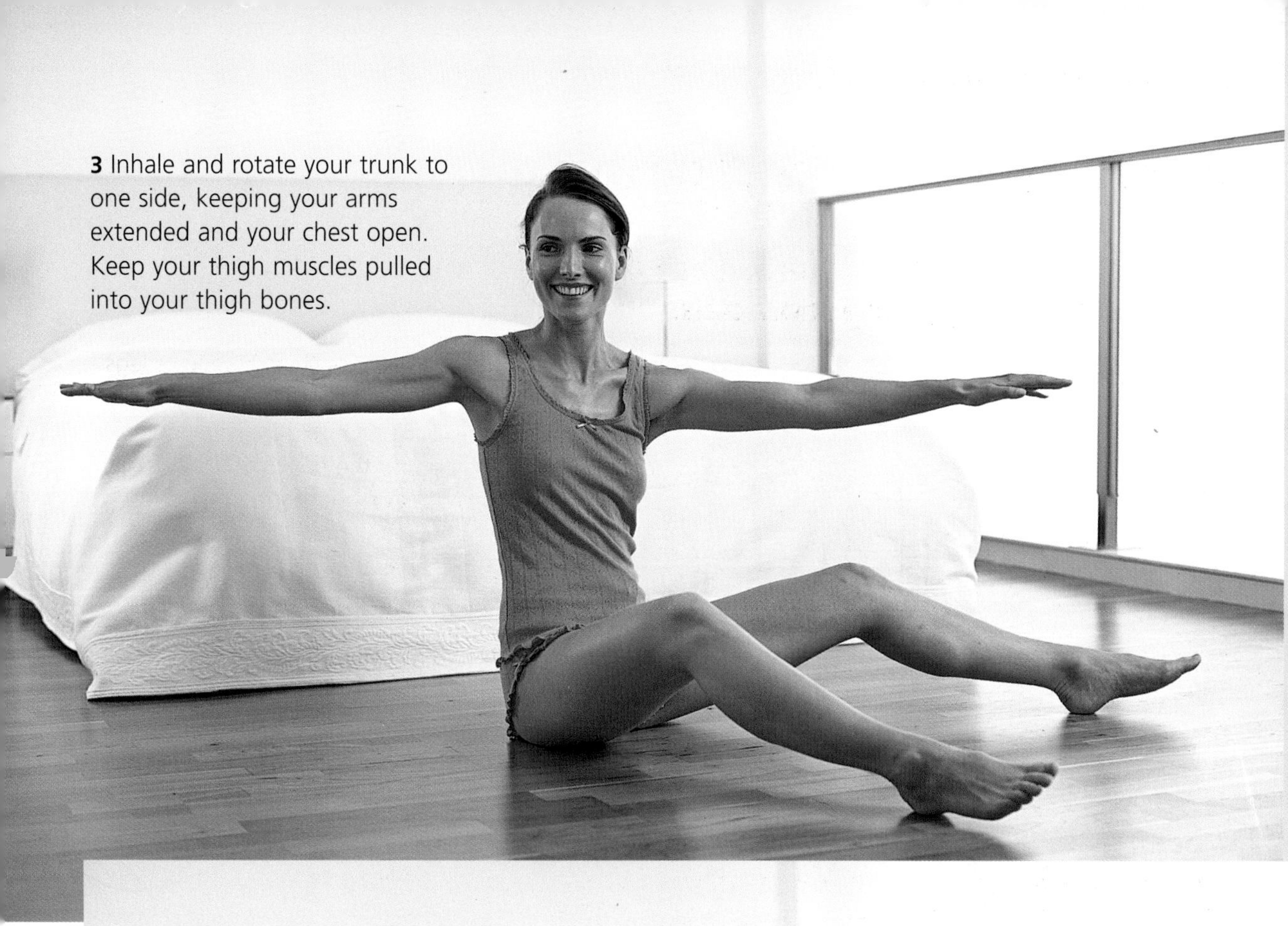

4 Exhale and lean forwards, stretching with one hand towards the big toe of your opposite foot, keeping your chest open and your armpits raised. Inhale then rotate your trunk back through the centre to the other side and, on the exhale, lean forwards and stretch towards the other foot. Perform 12 times on each side.

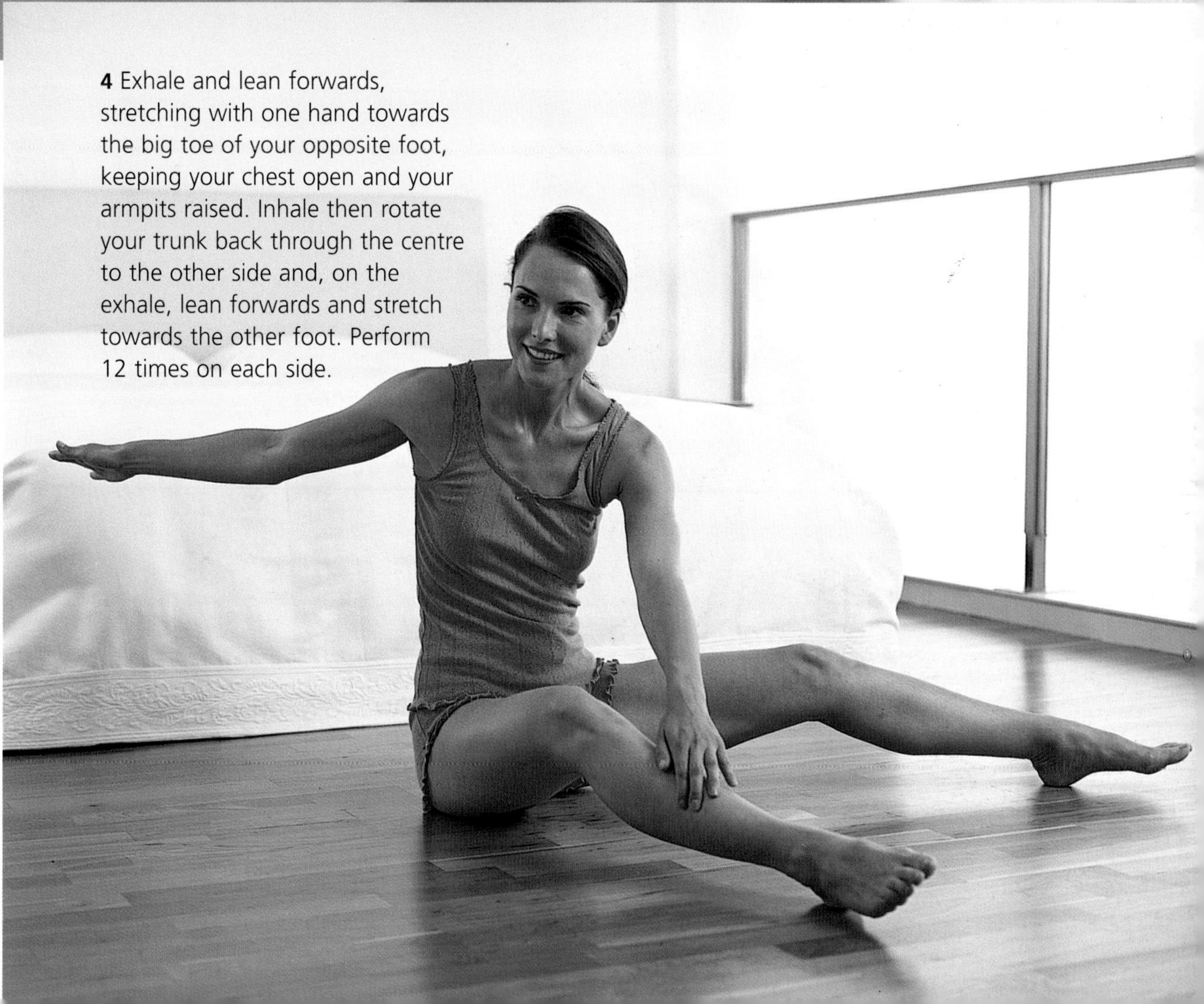

arm release

Release tension in the back of your upper arms with this stretch.

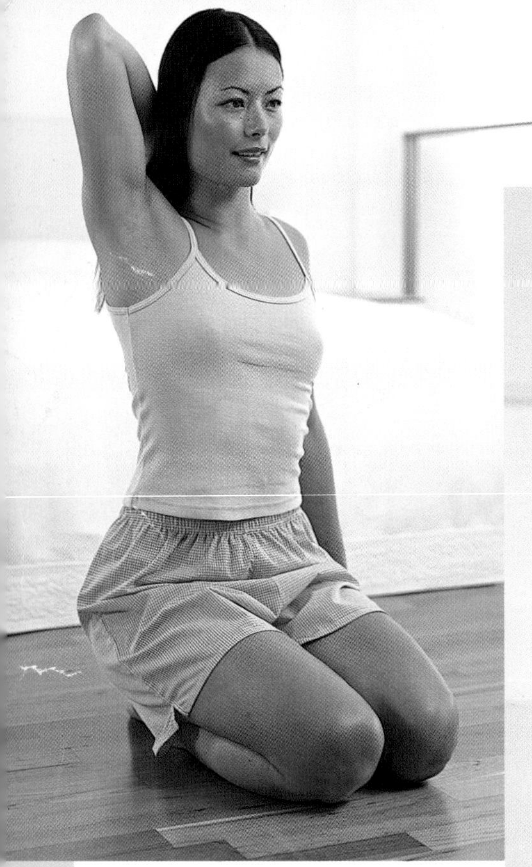

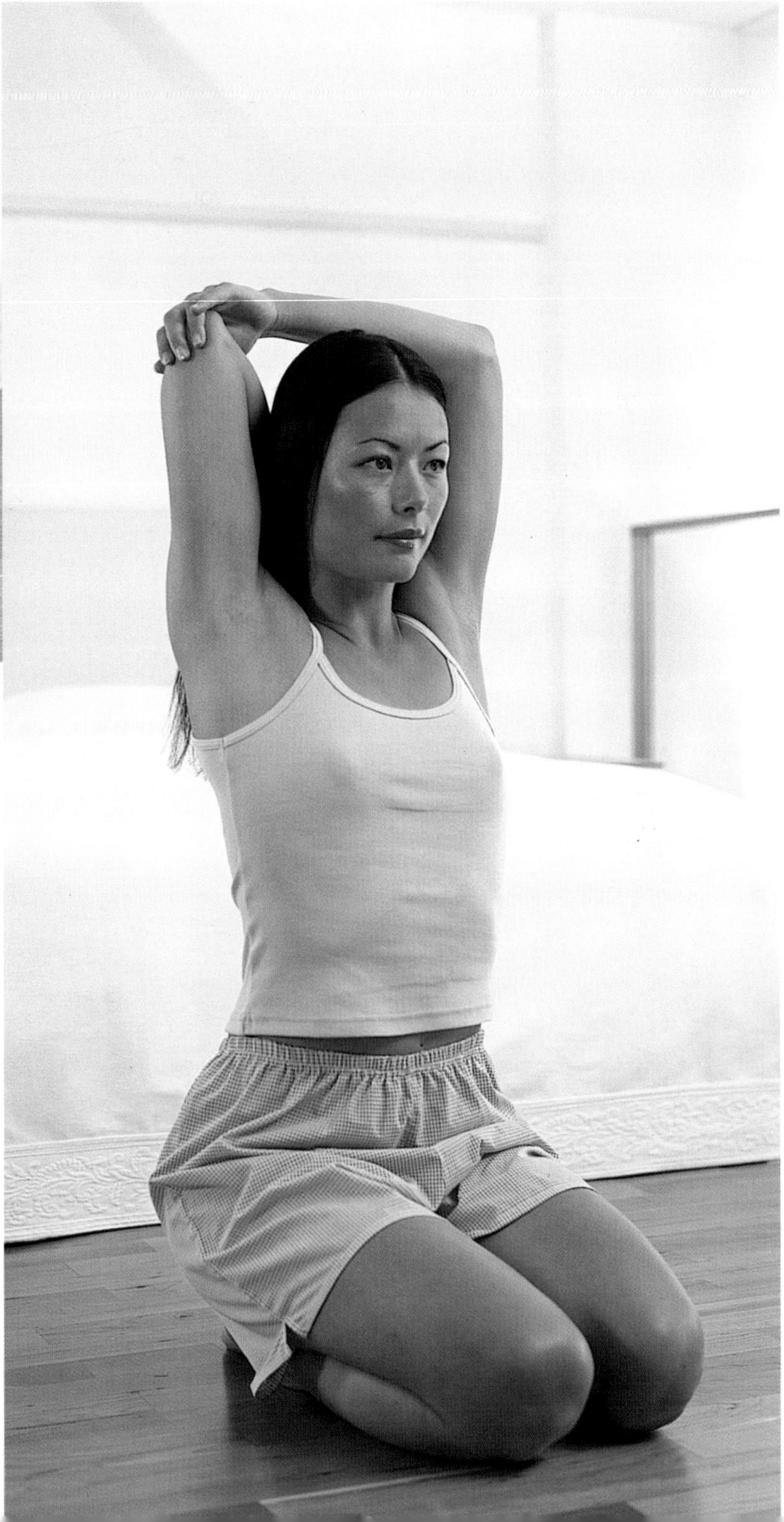

1 Adopt a kneeling position with your arms hanging down by your sides. Inhale and extend your right arm up above your head, then bend your elbow to drop your hand down between your shoulder blades and leave your elbow pointing upwards.

2 As you exhale place your left palm on your right elbow and ease your right arm further down your spine so as to stretch the triceps muscle. Hold for 3–5 breaths then repeat using the other arm.

side bends

These help increase your lateral movement strength, and also tone the waist and abdomen.

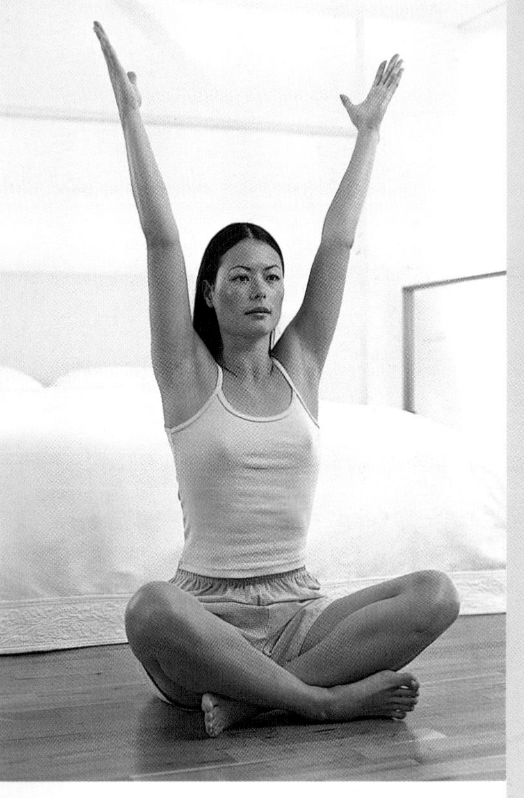

1 Sit cross-legged with your hips forwards. Take a deep breath to fill your lungs and open your rib cage. Hollow your abdomen by pulling it in towards your spine. Inhale and extend both arms above your head to elongate your spine.

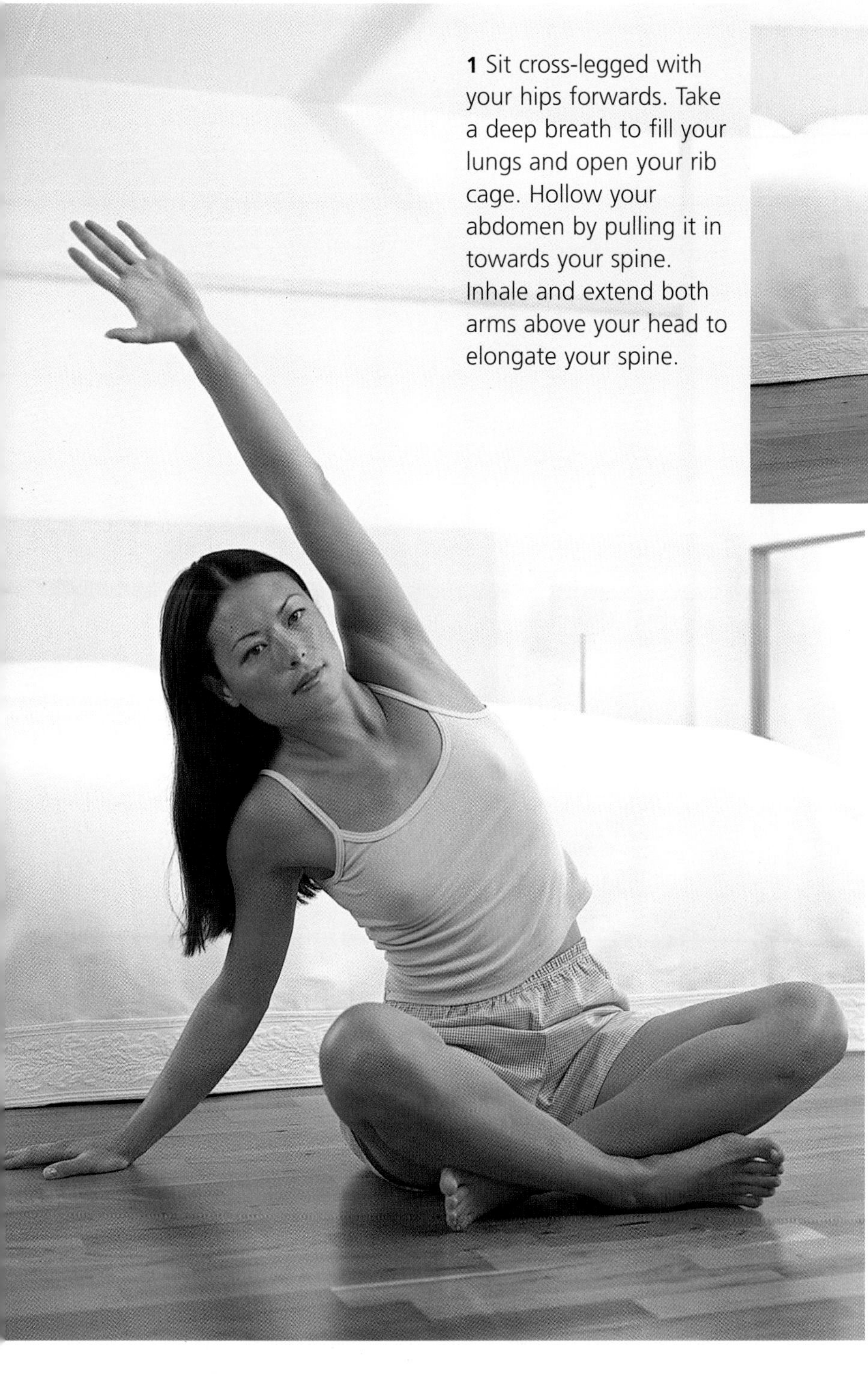

2 Exhale as you place your right palm on the floor and lean your trunk towards the right, extending your left arm over your head while keeping it close to your ear, so as to feel the stretch up the left side of your body. Keep your bottom flat on the floor and your abdomen hollow to stabilize your alignment. Inhale as you return to your starting position with both arms extended upwards. Exhale as you repeat the movement on the other side. Repeat the movement 5 times on each side, deepening your breathing and elongating your spine further each time.

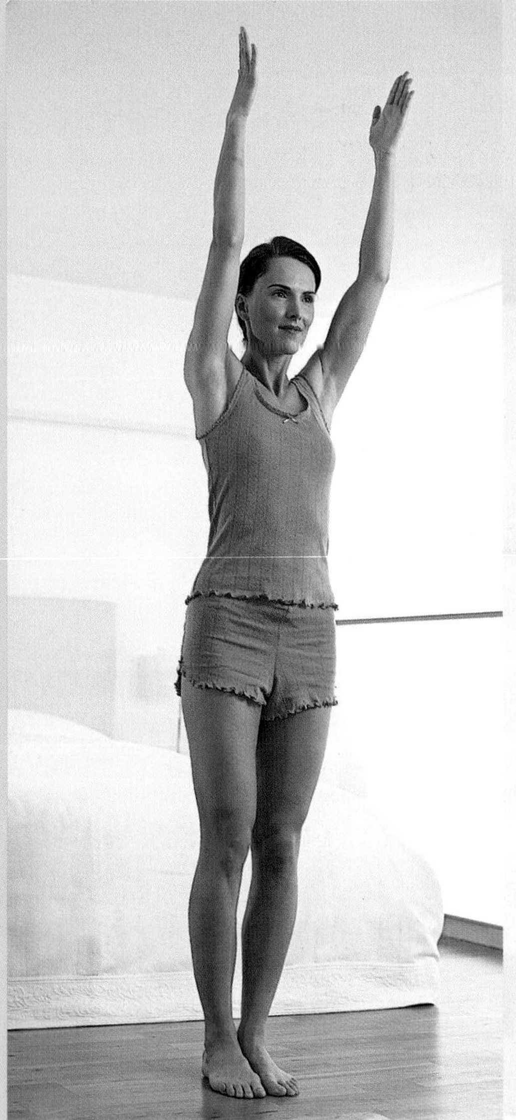

squats

These squats increase oxygen supply throughout the body to give you an early morning glow, and tone your buttocks and thighs.

1 Stand with your feet together and your weight evenly distributed. Pull your thigh muscles into your thigh bones. Keep your spine elongated, your abdomen hollow and your chest open. Your neck should be long and your shoulders down. Take a deep breath in to fill your rib cage and extend both your arms above your head.

2 As you exhale, step sideways to your right, keeping your spine long. Squat downwards, pushing your bottom and hips behind you as though about to sit down. At the same time pull your arms down and together in front of your trunk, your forearms facing you.

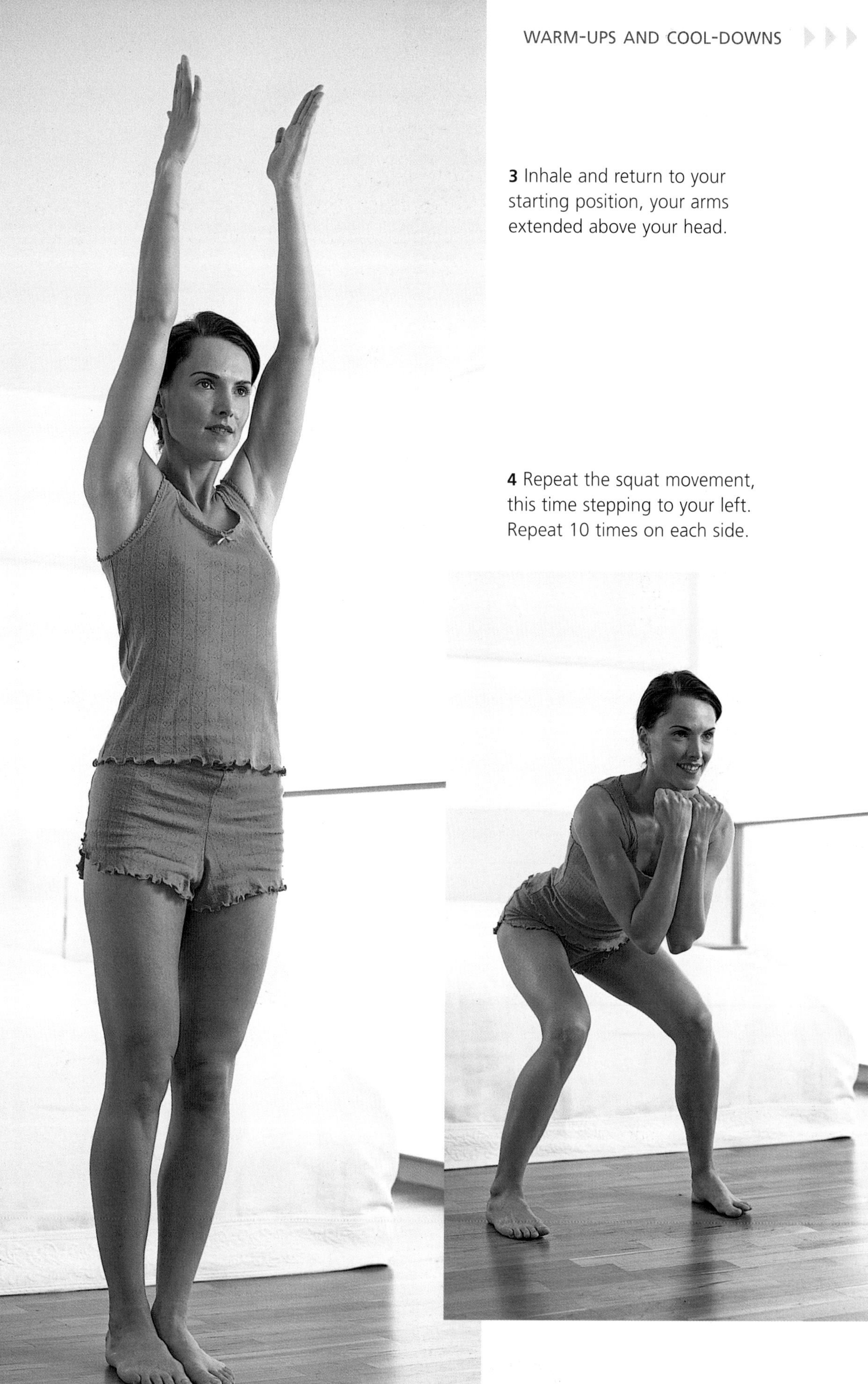

3 Inhale and return to your starting position, your arms extended above your head.

4 Repeat the squat movement, this time stepping to your left. Repeat 10 times on each side.

calf stretch

This is a good stretch for releasing tension in your lower legs.

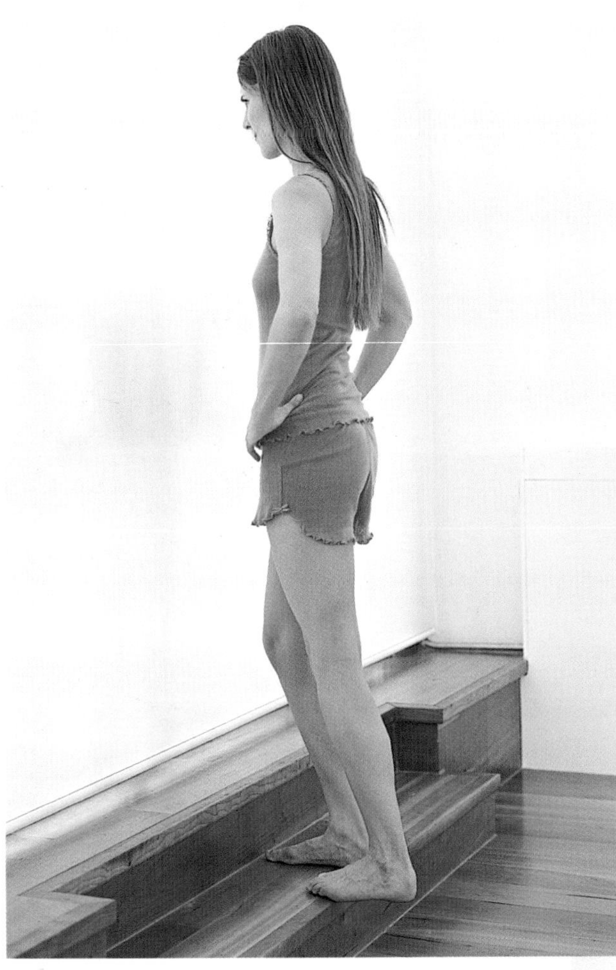

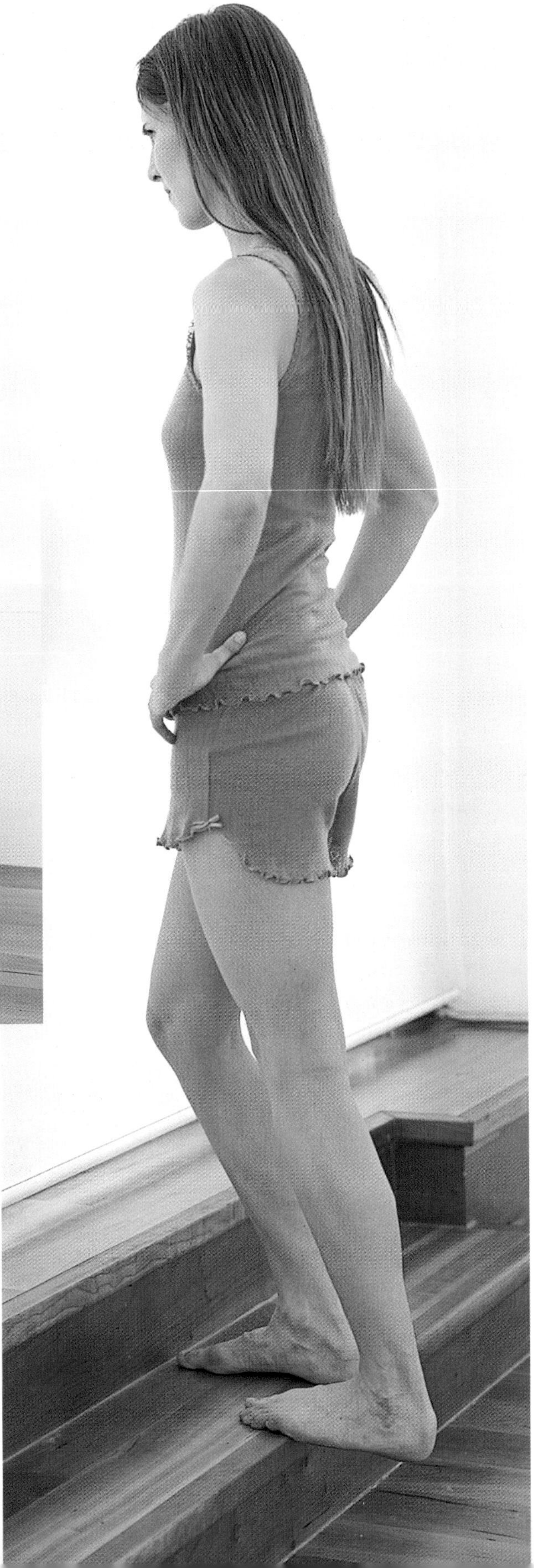

1 Stand on a step, bench or the bottom stair with your hands on your hips. Gently back the heel of your left foot off the edge of the platform.

2 Ensure you are standing erect. Inhale, then, as you exhale, gently press the heel of your left foot down towards the floor. Stop when you feel a gentle stretch in the back of your lower leg (your calf muscle). Hold for 5 cycles of slow breathing then repeat with the other foot.

trunk and spine release

This releases tension in the spine and trunk and is a good invigorating posture for starting the day.

1 Kneel down and lean forwards so as to rest your trunk on your elbows with your forearms flat on the floor in front of you. Your knees should be behind your hips and your elbows directly beneath your shoulders.

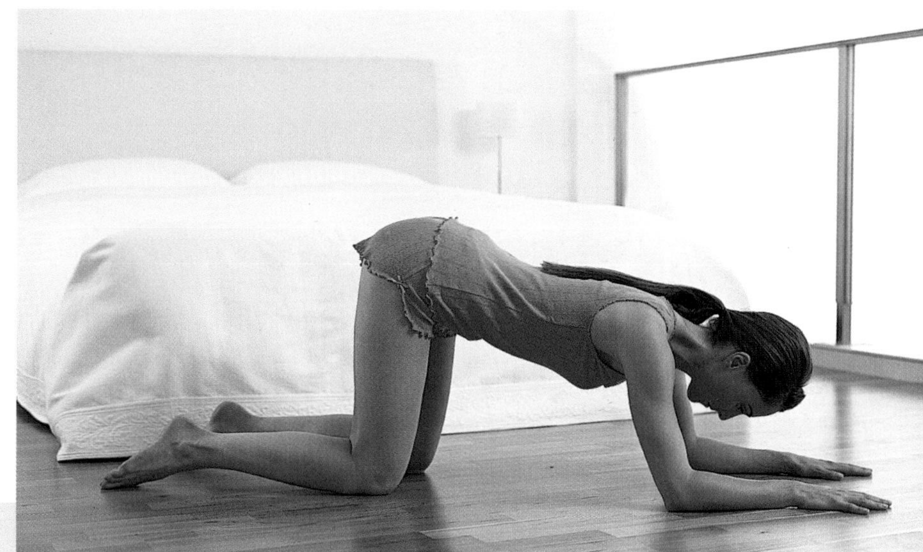

2 Bring your right palm towards your left elbow, inhale and stretch the left arm out of your trunk. As you exhale release your spine into the posture and drop your head on to your right forearm while maintaining downward and forward pressure in your left palm and arm. Hold for 10 cycles of breathing and then repeat with the other arm.

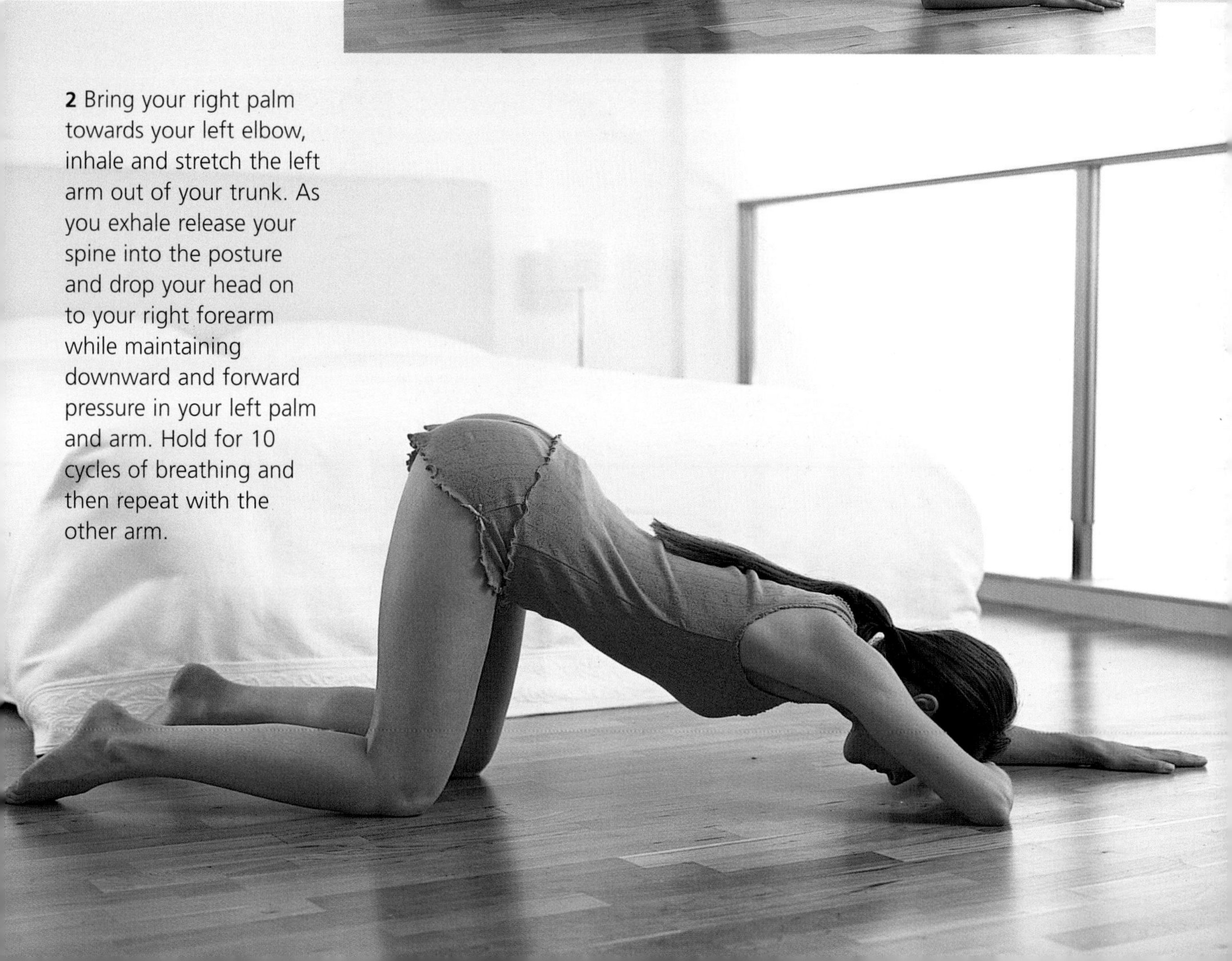

hamstring lengthener

This yoga-inspired position strengthens the spine and improves posture while elongating the backs of your legs.

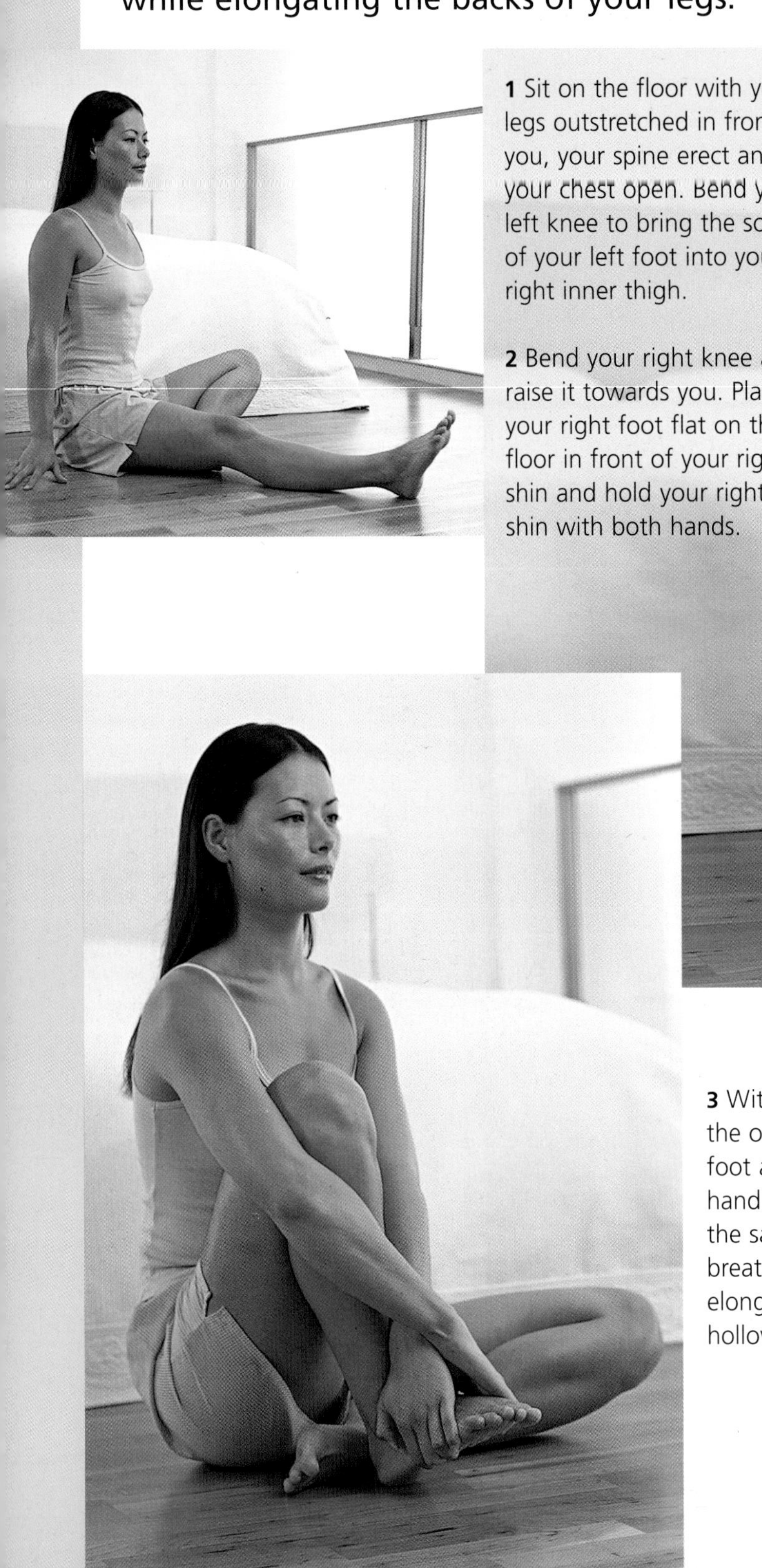

1 Sit on the floor with your legs outstretched in front of you, your spine erect and your chest open. Bend your left knee to bring the sole of your left foot into your right inner thigh.

2 Bend your right knee and raise it towards you. Place your right foot flat on the floor in front of your right shin and hold your right shin with both hands.

3 With your left hand grip the outer edge of your right foot and with your right hand grip the inner edge of the same foot. Take a deep breath to fill your rib cage, elongate your spine and hollow your abdomen.

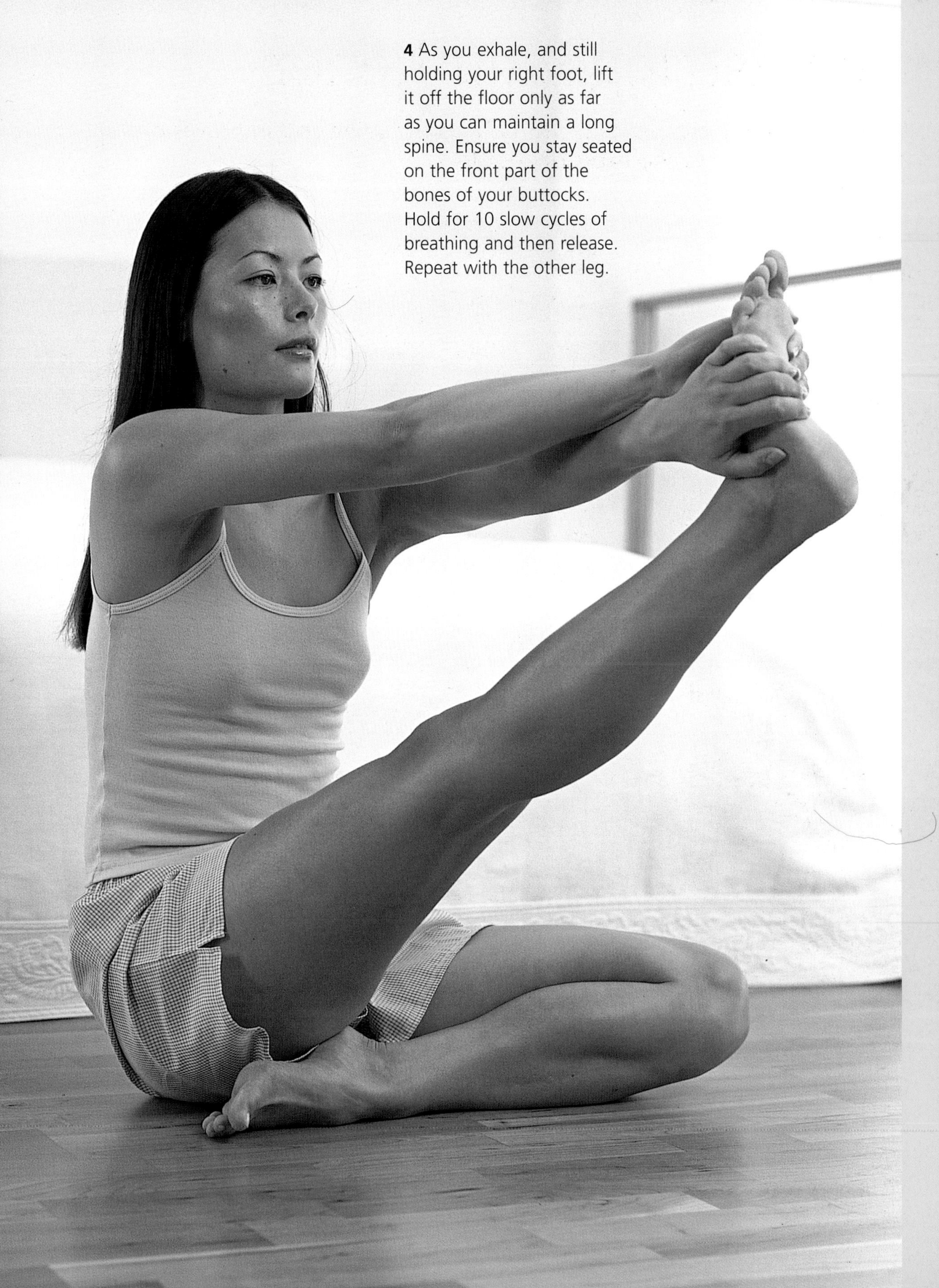

4 As you exhale, and still holding your right foot, lift it off the floor only as far as you can maintain a long spine. Ensure you stay seated on the front part of the bones of your buttocks. Hold for 10 slow cycles of breathing and then release. Repeat with the other leg.

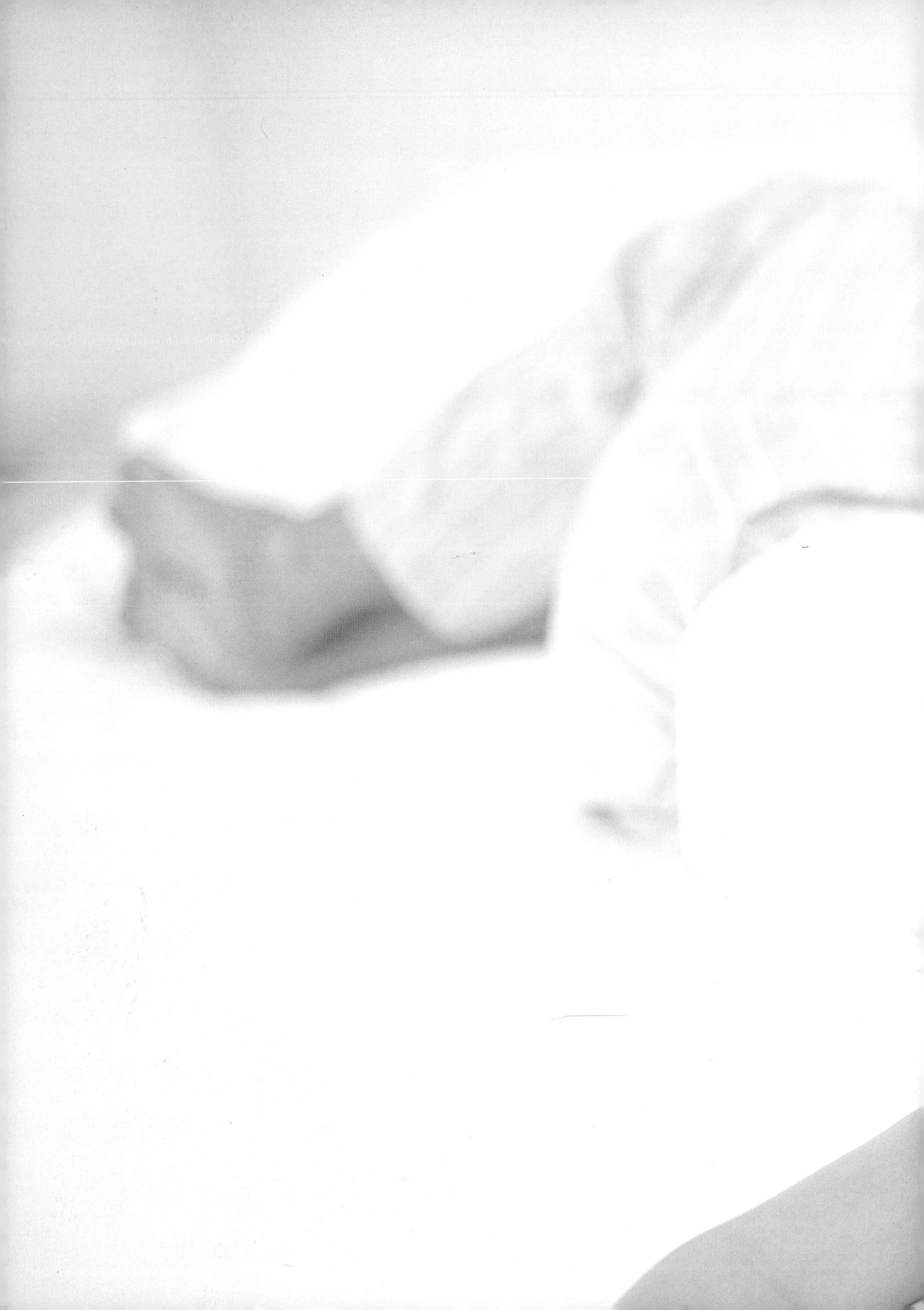

rise and shine

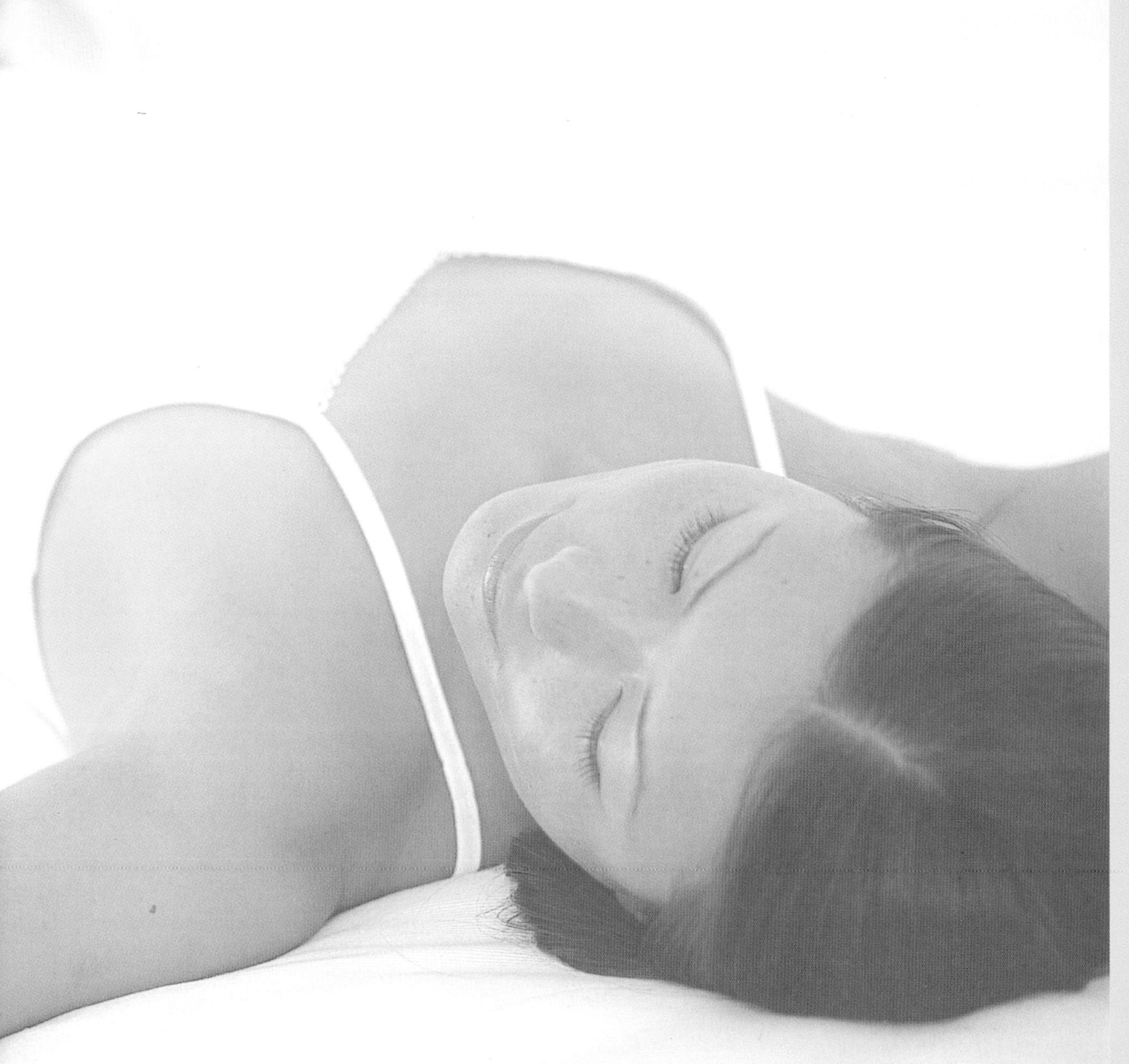

rise and shine

One of the easiest workouts to practise, this is the best one to try once you have mastered the warm-ups and cool-downs. Some of the exercises can actually be performed in bed – you don't even have to get up to tone your thighs, strengthen your legs and arms and release tension in your spine! Others are for performing in the bathroom during your bathing routine and will help you to improve your strength and fitness for the other workouts.

Wake up with water

Hydrotherapy techniques use the power of water to revitalize your energy systems and are especially useful for mornings when you have to drag yourself out of bed. They will leave you totally energized and ready to start the day.

Eye splashing

This quick wake-up call freshens and increases circulation and colour to the face. Bend over the bathroom basin and run the tap with fairly cool water. Inhale, then as you exhale cup your hands under the water and splash your face seven times with your eyes open. Immediately dry your face and moisturize.

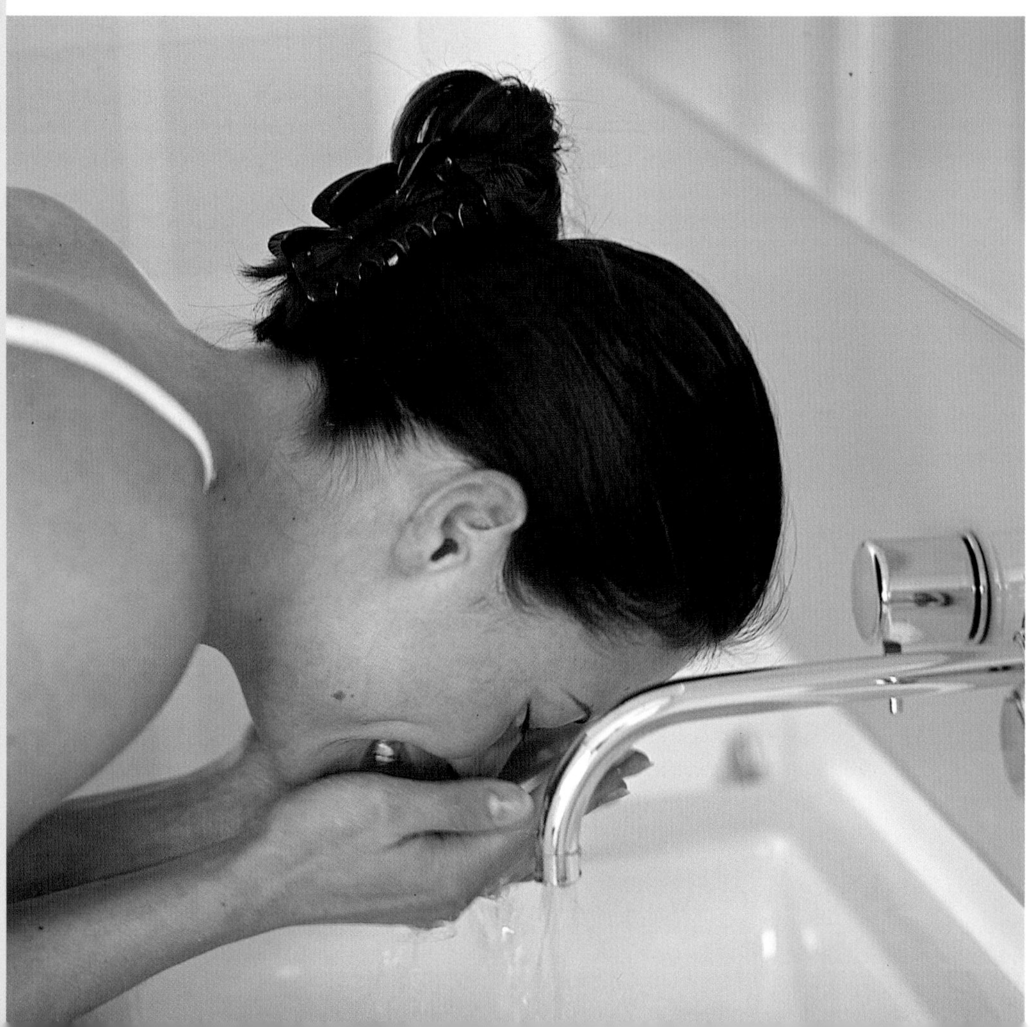

BRIGHT EYES

If you often wake with tired and puffy eyes keep a flask of hot water by your bed so that you can drink a glass of it first thing, then lie back in bed for 10 minutes. The hot water helps to kick-start your kidneys and release retained water from the delicate tissue around the eyes. As you lie back focus your mind so that you become aware of your breathing, without altering the natural flow of your breath.

'Some of the exercises can be performed in bed – so you don't even have to get up to tone and strengthen your body'

Shower power

Invigorating jets of water are ideal for getting the blood pumping. If you're brave enough, vary the temperature in your shower for a quick pep-up. The contrast of hot and cold water will tone you up, get the circulation going, stimulate your internal organs, boost your immune system and leave your whole body tingling with pleasure and raring to go. Start the shower warm, then turn the temperature down as cool as you can bear for 30 seconds, then turn it back up. Repeat this two or three times, finishing with a cold blast. Wrap yourself up in warm towels, pat yourself dry and rest for a few minutes, before channelling your newfound energy into a quick burst of exercise.

Spritz awake

There will be occasional days when you won't want to wake up, let alone work out, so try a quick spritz of soothing essential oils to invigorate yourself and help you combat headaches, muscle tension, anxiety and burn-out symptoms. There are some excellent products and sprays on the market or you can buy an atomizer and create your own blend of oils.

Lavender is a versatile and gentle essence, which relieves the above symptoms and combines well with other oils like sandalwood and geranium for instant relaxation. Specific ailments treatable with other essential oils include headaches (basil, eucalyptus, peppermint), burn-out (bergamot, rosemary), migraine (camomile, peppermint), muscle tension (camomile, clary sage, rosemary) and anxiety (clary sage, melissa, neroli, rosewood, patchouli). Some essential oils can have adverse effects if you are pregnant, so always consult a qualified aromatherapist first.

Carry your oil or blend of oils around with you in your bag and spritz your temples, earlobes or the insides of your wrists when necessary. Combine with a gentle massage of your temples or the back of your neck for extra relief. Alternatively, put a couple of drops of your chosen oils on a handkerchief and take a deep inhalation whenever you need a quick-fix or instant stress buster.

revitalizing breathing

Help rejuvenate your circulation and gently awaken your body with this calming breathing exercise.

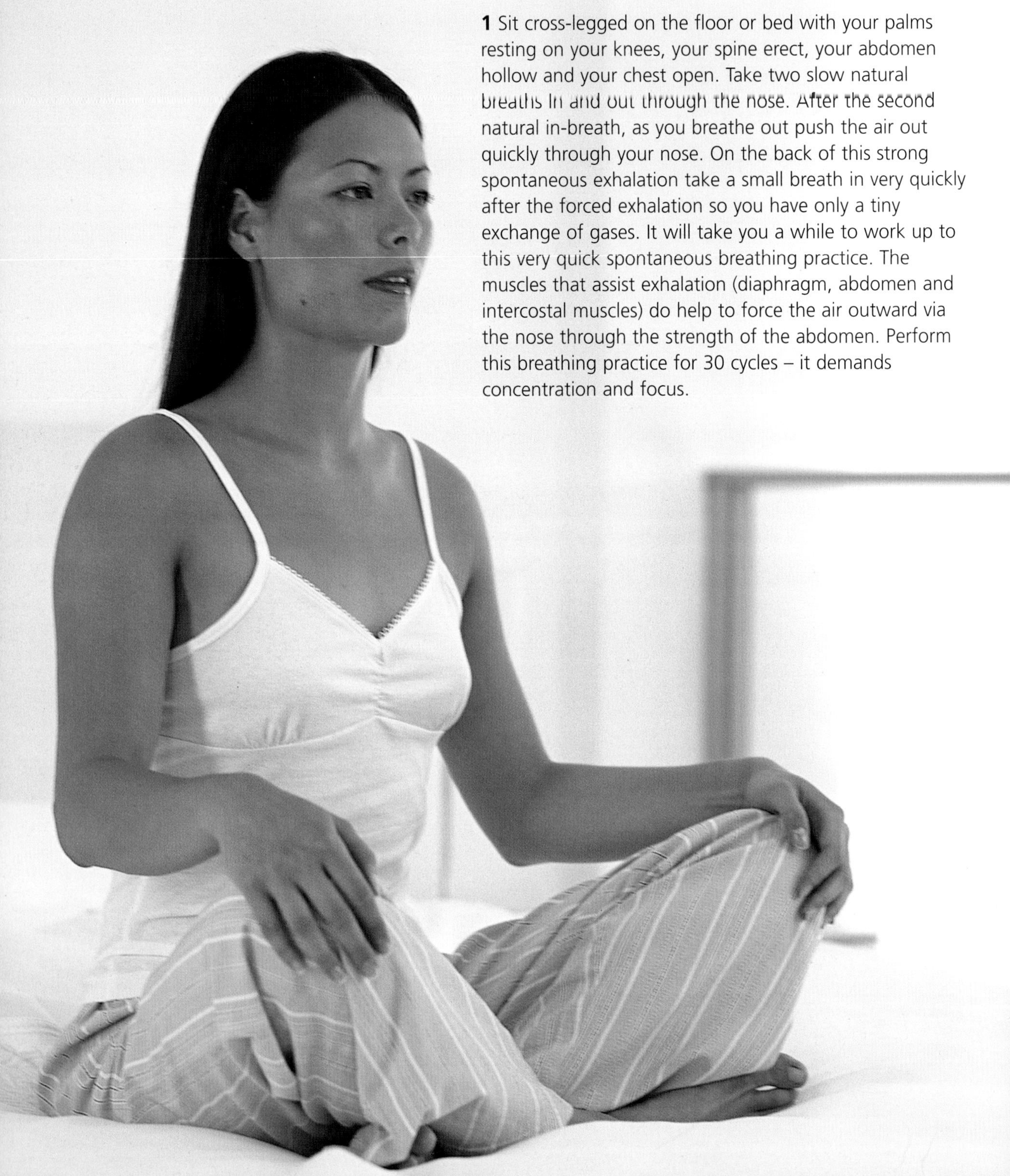

1 Sit cross-legged on the floor or bed with your palms resting on your knees, your spine erect, your abdomen hollow and your chest open. Take two slow natural breaths in and out through the nose. After the second natural in-breath, as you breathe out push the air out quickly through your nose. On the back of this strong spontaneous exhalation take a small breath in very quickly after the forced exhalation so you have only a tiny exchange of gases. It will take you a while to work up to this very quick spontaneous breathing practice. The muscles that assist exhalation (diaphragm, abdomen and intercostal muscles) do help to force the air outward via the nose through the strength of the abdomen. Perform this breathing practice for 30 cycles – it demands concentration and focus.

easy spinal twist

This stretch releases the tension that builds up in your spine and pelvis while you are asleep and static in bed.

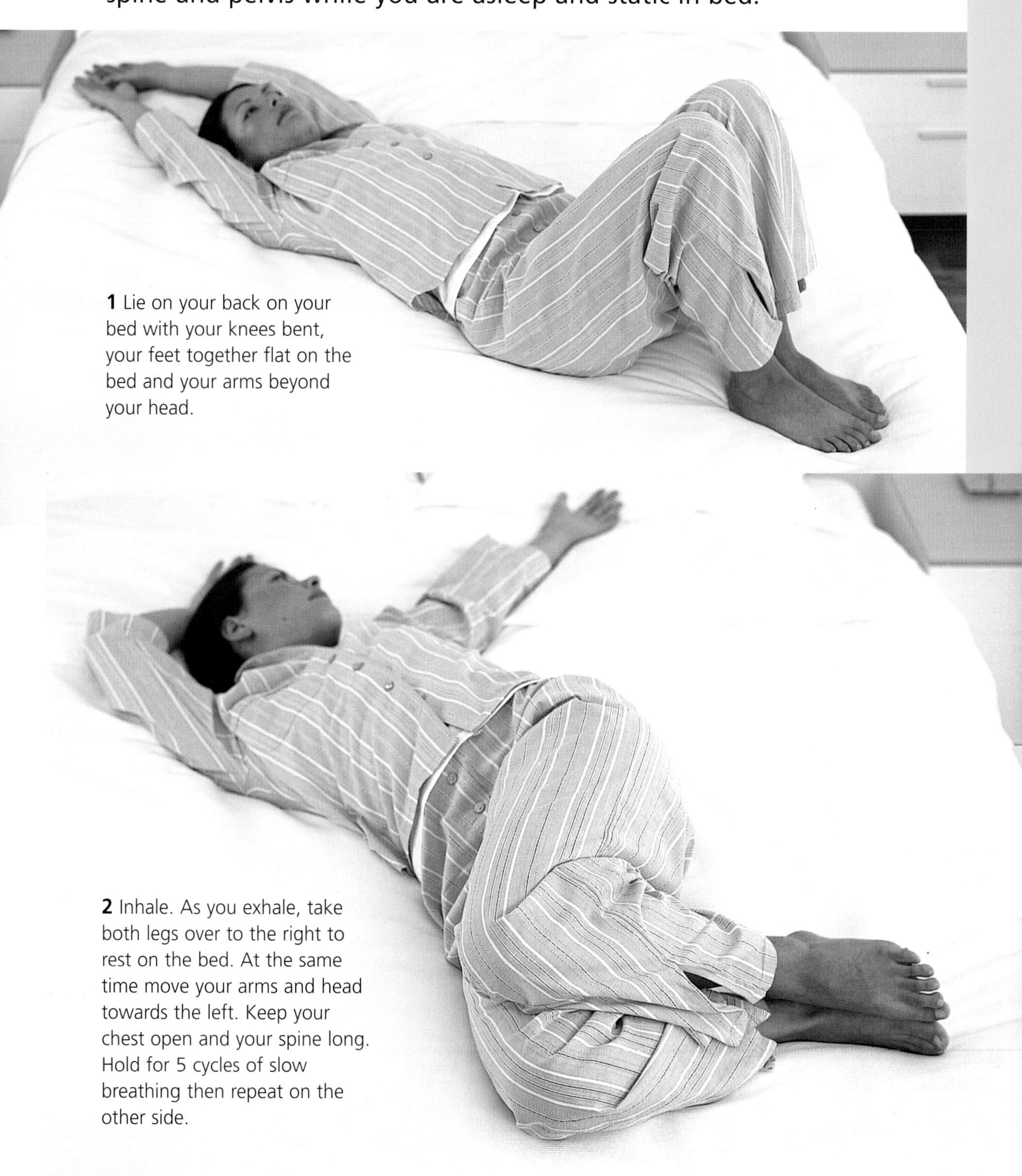

1 Lie on your back on your bed with your knees bent, your feet together flat on the bed and your arms beyond your head.

2 Inhale. As you exhale, take both legs over to the right to rest on the bed. At the same time move your arms and head towards the left. Keep your chest open and your spine long. Hold for 5 cycles of slow breathing then repeat on the other side.

butterfly pelvis release

This releases tension in your hips and your lumbar spine – a useful exercise if you spend much time sitting.

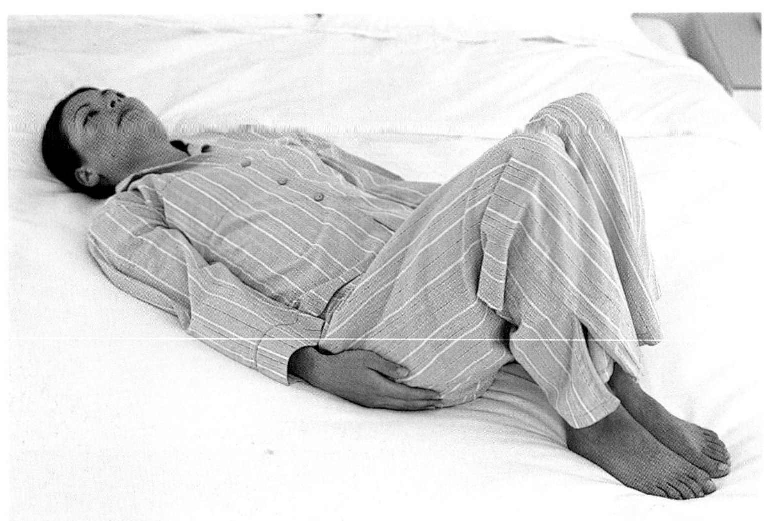

1 Lie on your back on your bed with your knees bent, your feet together flat on the bed and your hands by your sides with your chest open.

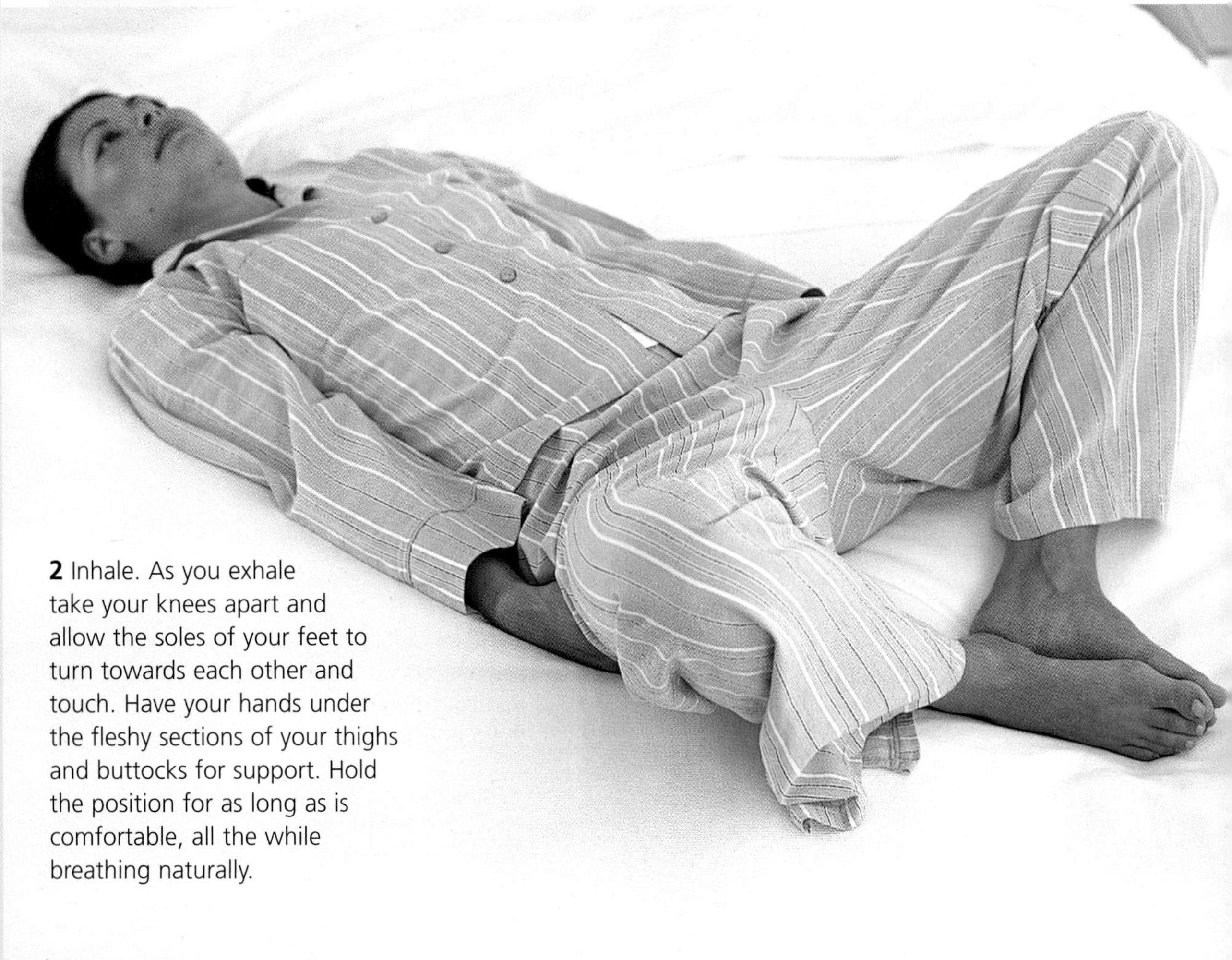

2 Inhale. As you exhale take your knees apart and allow the soles of your feet to turn towards each other and touch. Have your hands under the fleshy sections of your thighs and buttocks for support. Hold the position for as long as is comfortable, all the while breathing naturally.

reverse child pose

This classic posture releases tension in your lower spine and shoulders. It also helps to relax the hip and neck muscles.

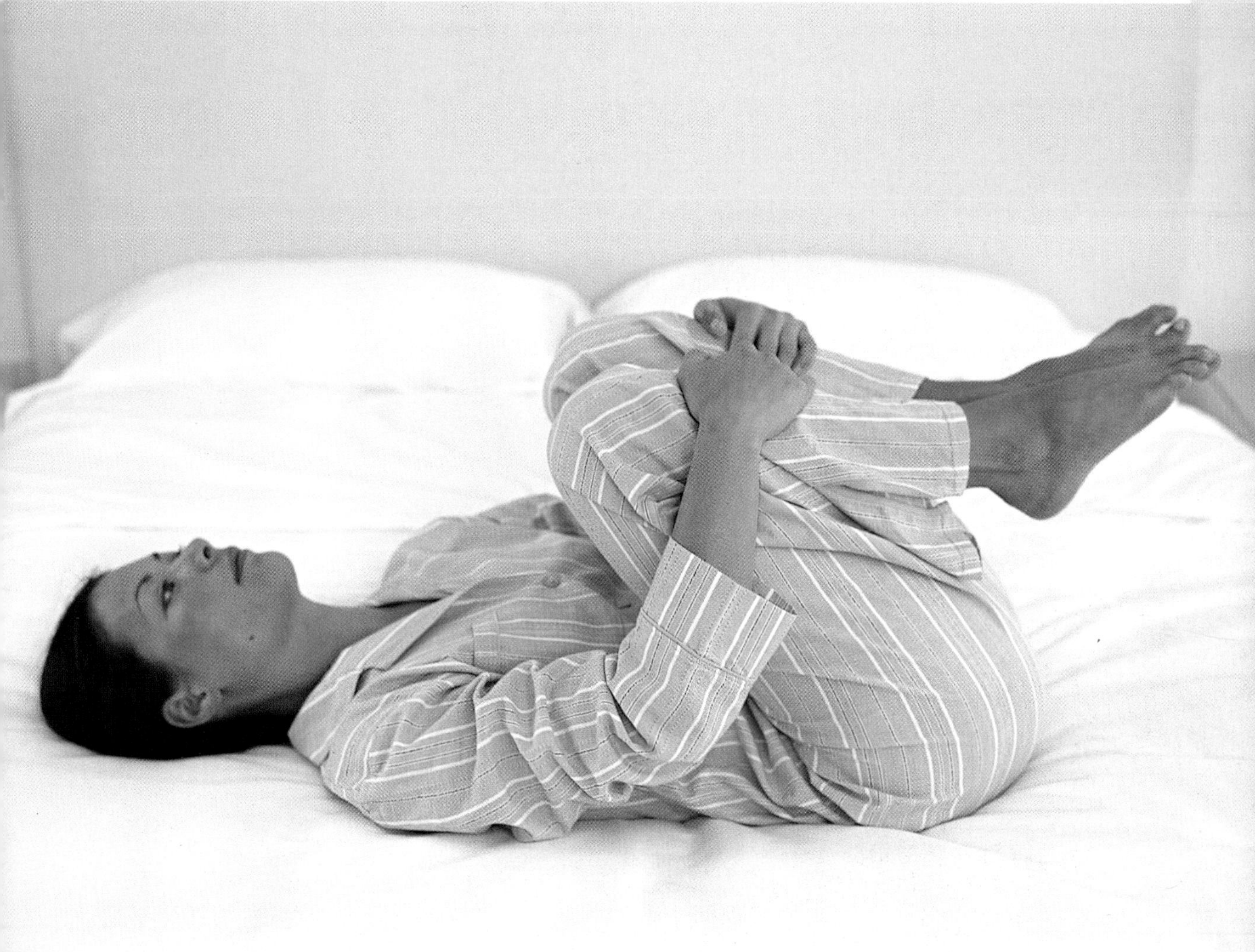

1 Lie on your back on your bed with your legs bent and your feet flat on the bed. Take a deep breath to fill your rib cage. As you exhale, bring both legs towards you, holding your shins to help your knees come forwards towards your chest. If you have knee problems, hold your legs behind your thighs. Breathe deeply and slowly for 3–5 breaths. Release.

spine awakener

This is great for opening the spine and stretching your trunk muscles. This exercise offers three levels of difficulty. Do not work beyond step 2 (gentle) if you have a prolapsed disc or back injury.

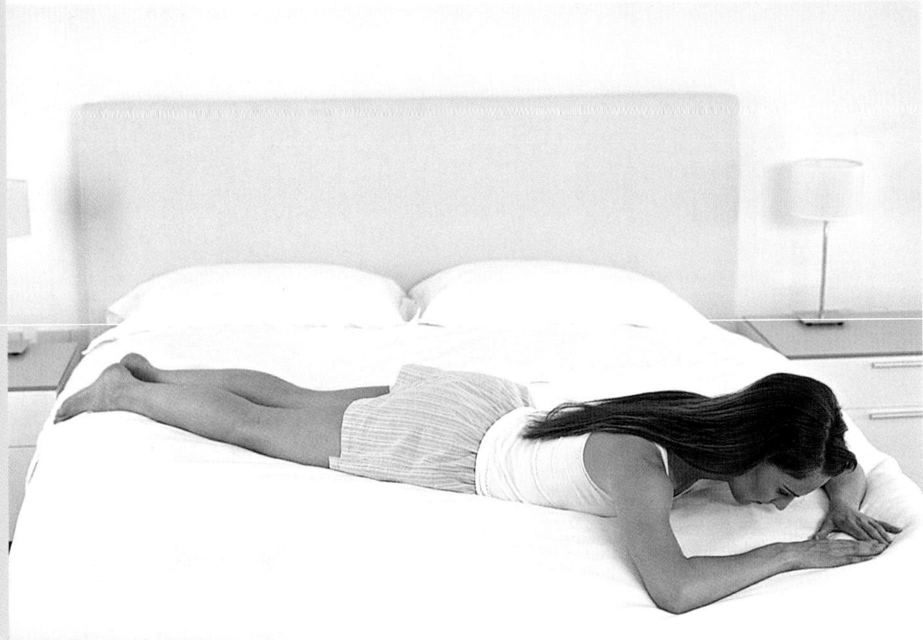

1 Lie on your front on the bed with your legs together, your elbows pointing out to the sides and your palms flat on the bed. Pull your abdomen in towards your spine and ensure your neck is long and away from your shoulders.

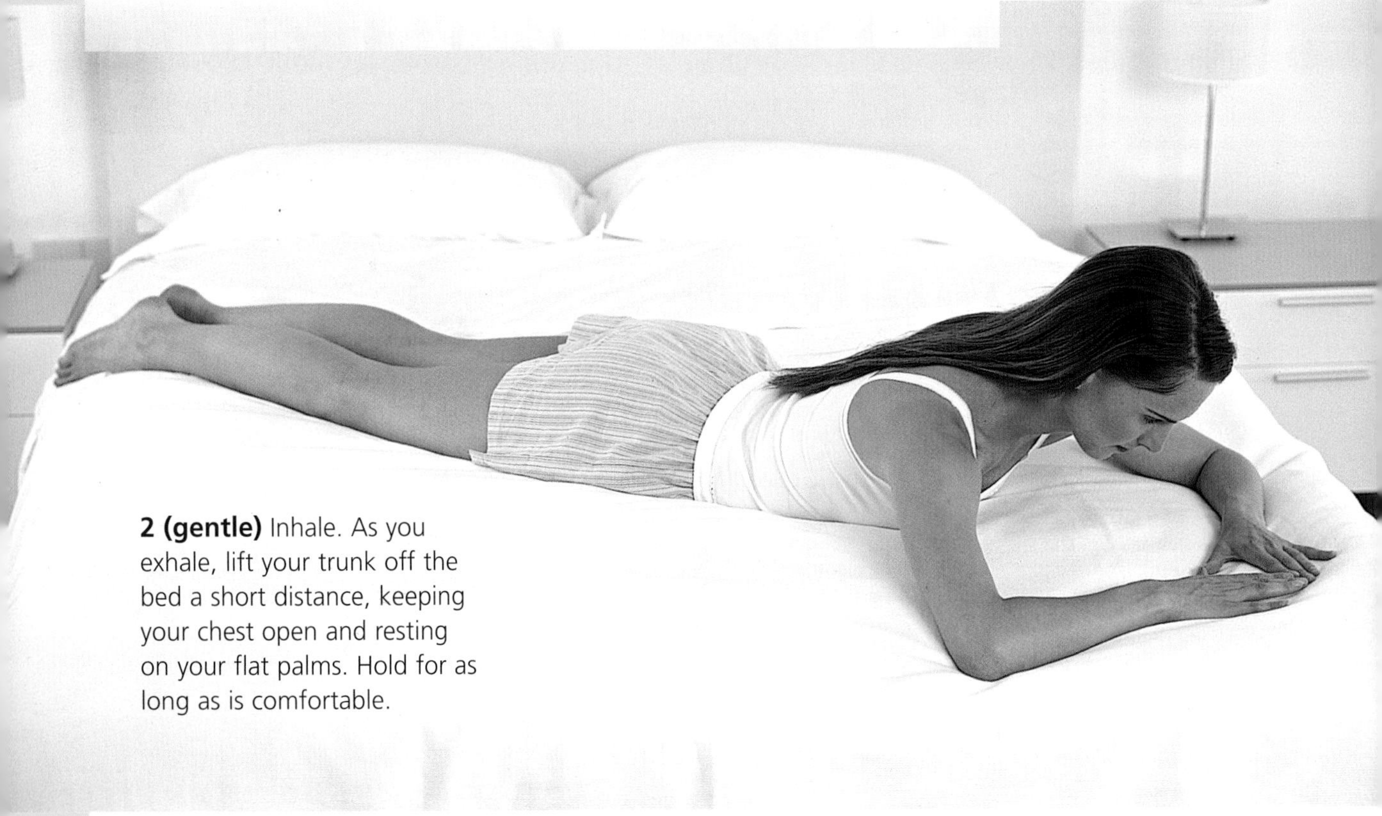

2 (gentle) Inhale. As you exhale, lift your trunk off the bed a short distance, keeping your chest open and resting on your flat palms. Hold for as long as is comfortable.

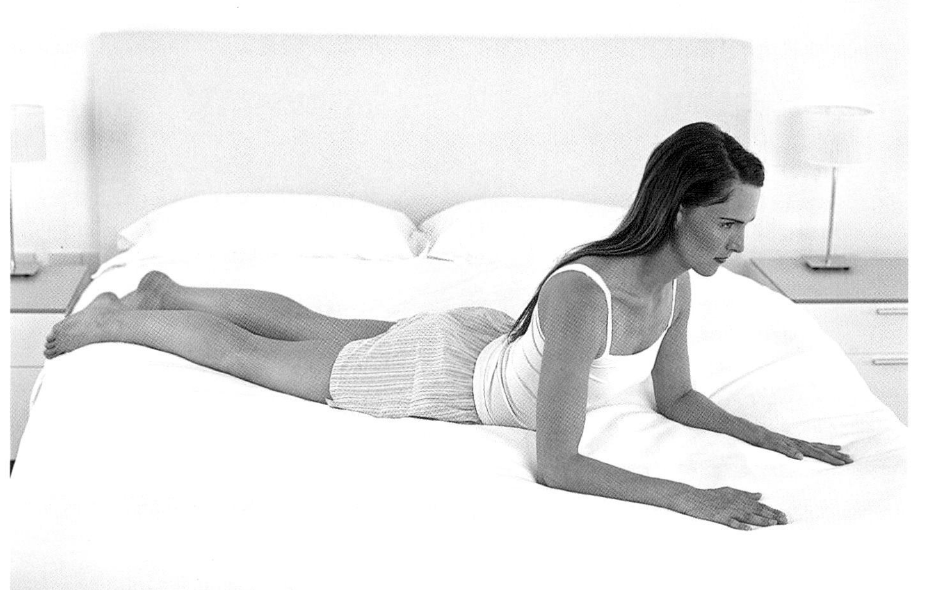

2 (moderate) To make the exercise more challenging, inhale and bring your forearms in front of you so as to prop up your trunk on your elbows.

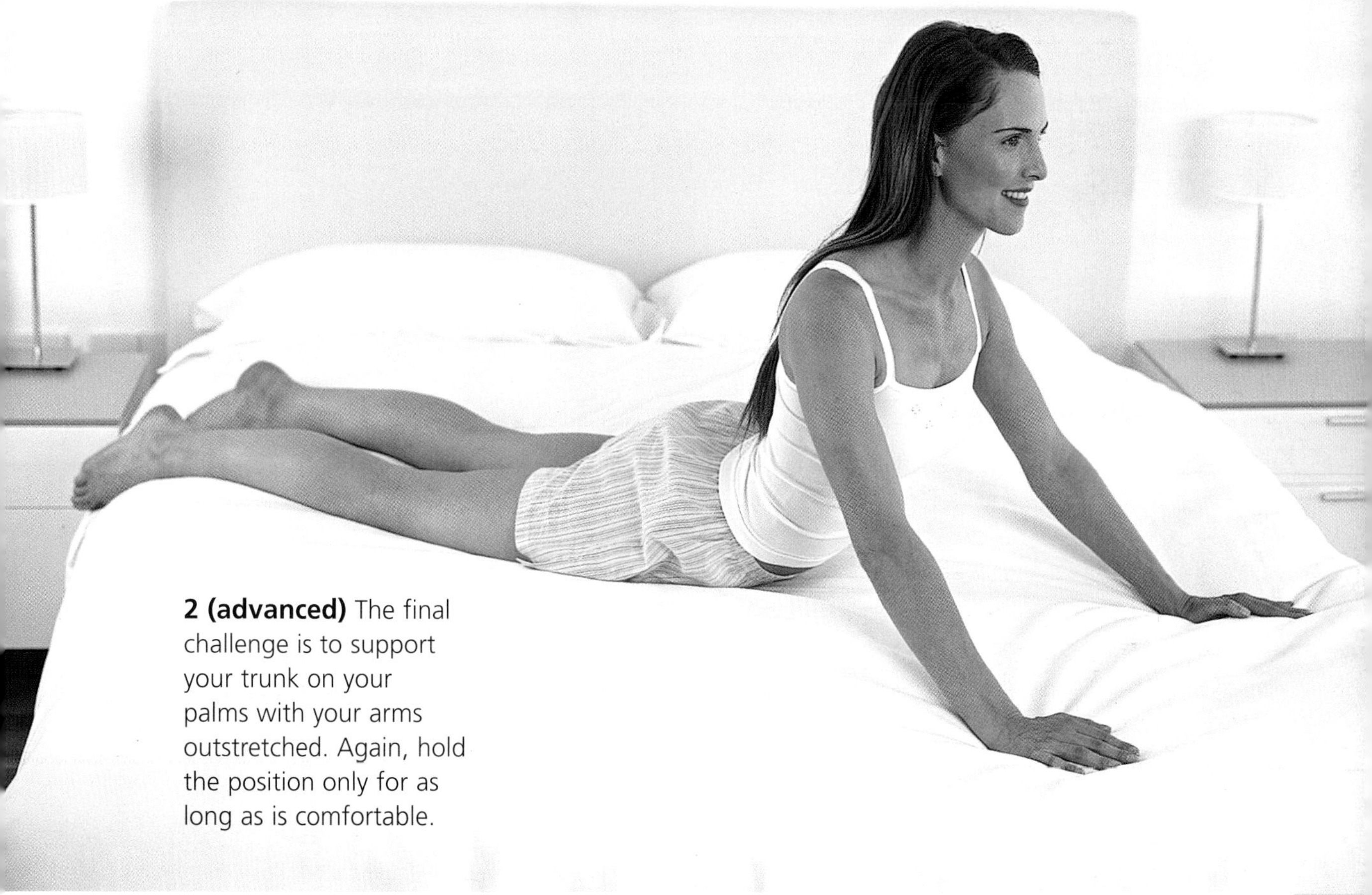

2 (advanced) The final challenge is to support your trunk on your palms with your arms outstretched. Again, hold the position only for as long as is comfortable.

seated bed twists

These movements tone the waist and abdominals while maintaining healthy intervertebral discs in your spine.

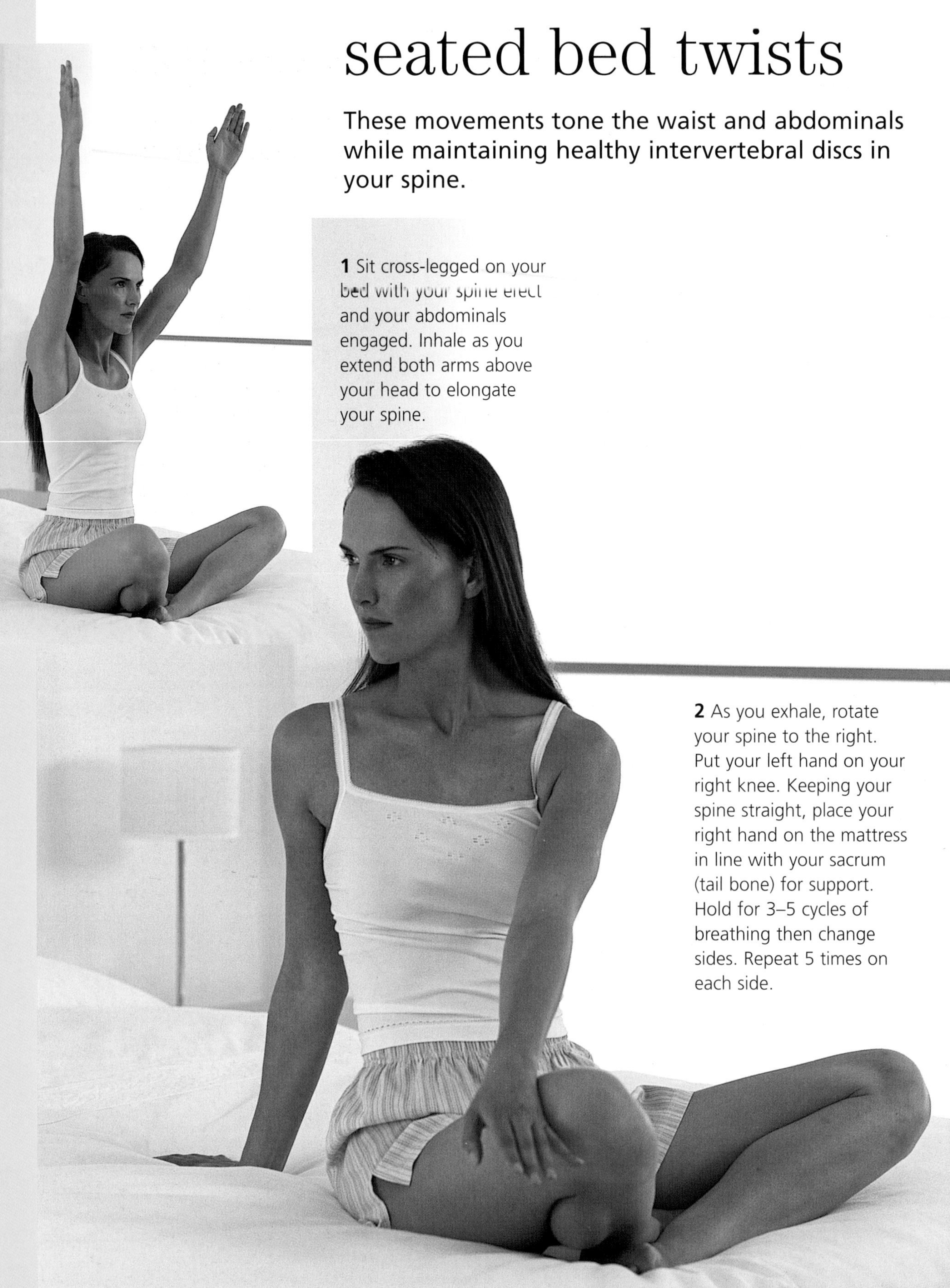

1 Sit cross-legged on your bed with your spine erect and your abdominals engaged. Inhale as you extend both arms above your head to elongate your spine.

2 As you exhale, rotate your spine to the right. Put your left hand on your right knee. Keeping your spine straight, place your right hand on the mattress in line with your sacrum (tail bone) for support. Hold for 3–5 cycles of breathing then change sides. Repeat 5 times on each side.

spine roll wake-ups

This is perfect for releasing spinal tension and it also stretches your legs. If you can't touch the floor easily with your hands, bend your knees to support your spine.

1 Stand with your feet hip width apart, your hips level and your weight evenly distributed on your feet. Draw your thigh muscles into your thigh bones. Your sacrum (tail bone) should be tucked inwards slightly. Keep your shoulders relaxed and your neck long, away from your shoulders. Take a deep breath to fill your rib cage, expanding this area as much as is comfortable.

2 As you exhale, engage your abdominals and begin to lean forwards. 'Roll' your spine downwards, moving slowly all the way until you are bending right over as far as is comfortable. Rest. Inhale. As you exhale begin to roll your spine gently back up to your starting position. Be careful to maintain the length you gain from the spine roll, growing taller into the space above your head. Repeat 5 times.

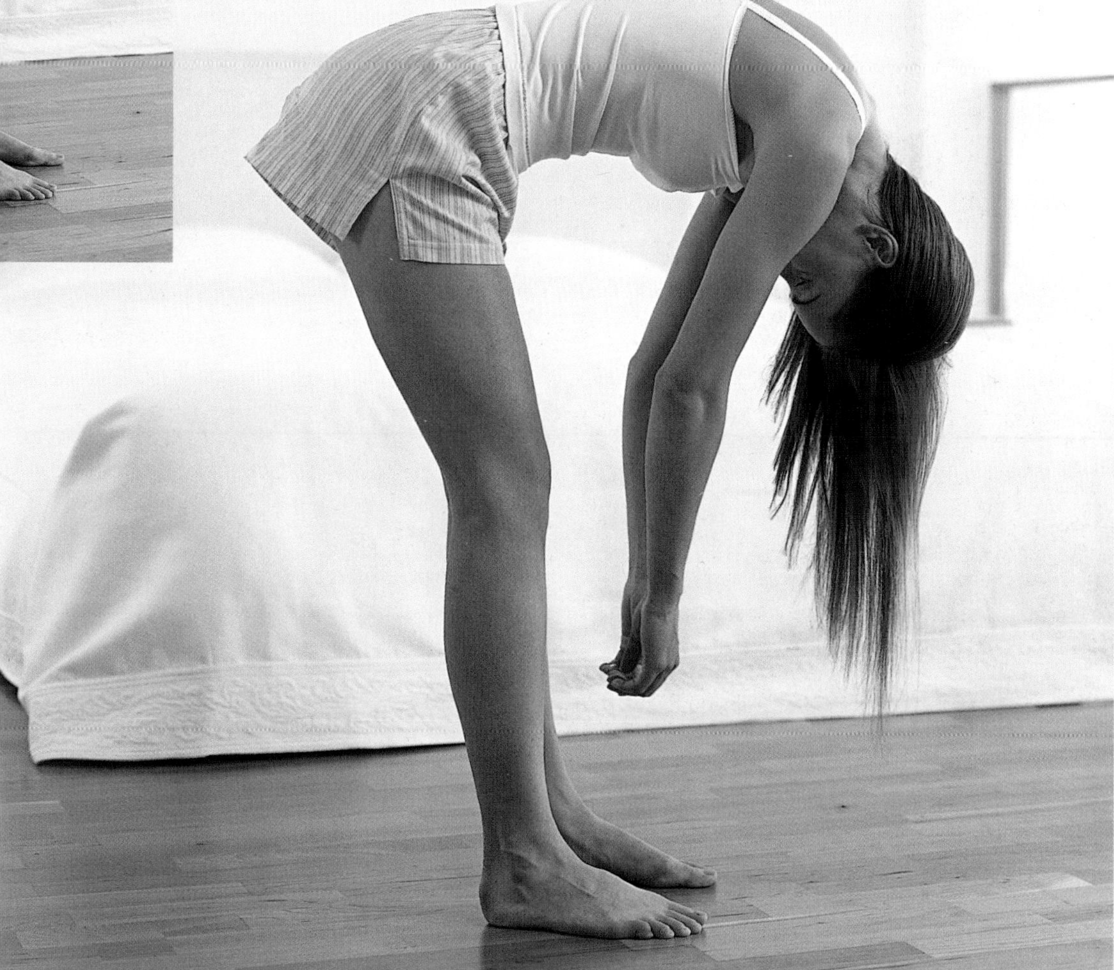

shoulder rotators

This is especially good for mobilizing the shoulder joints and toning the upper arms.

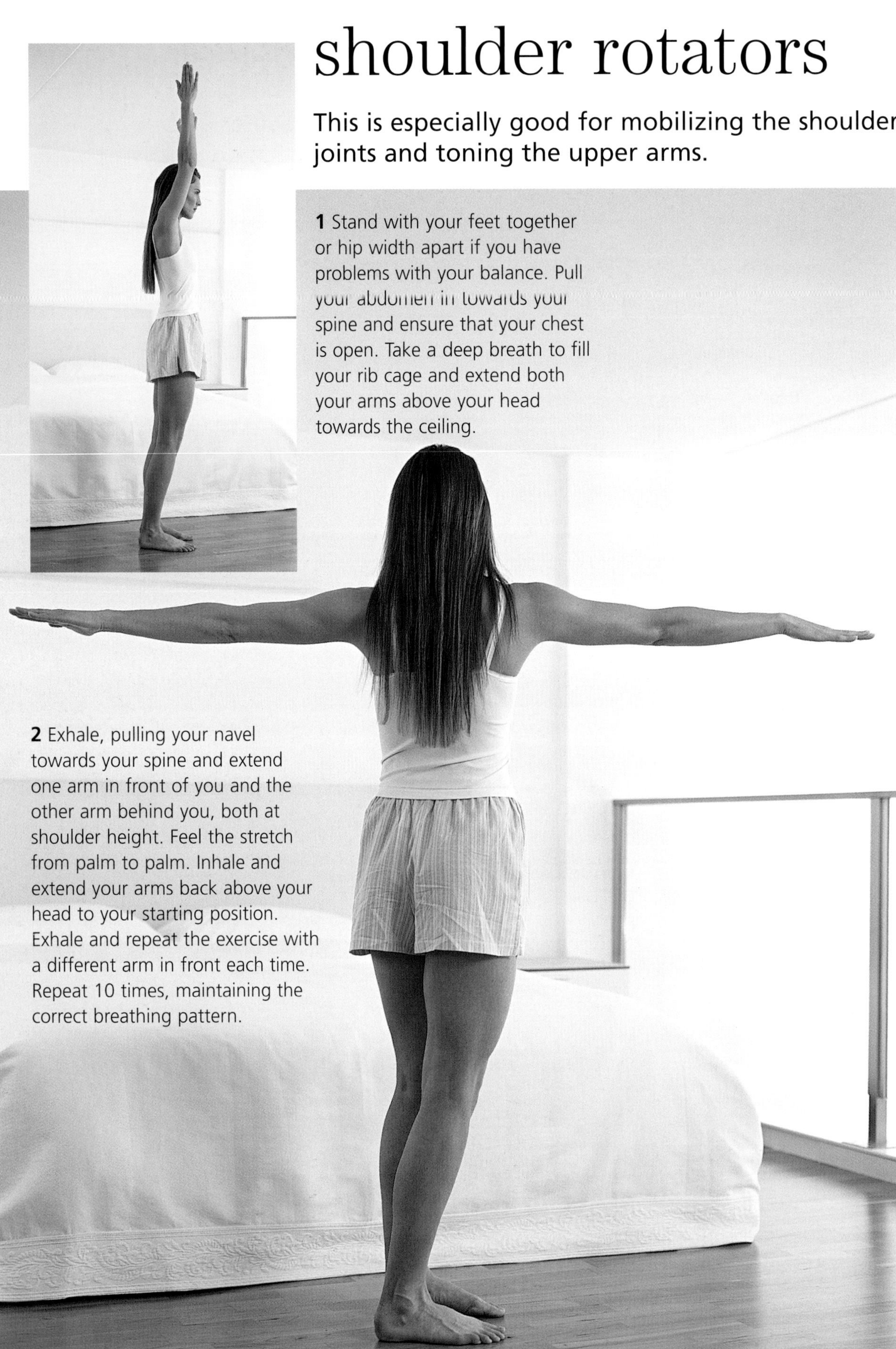

1 Stand with your feet together or hip width apart if you have problems with your balance. Pull your abdomen in towards your spine and ensure that your chest is open. Take a deep breath to fill your rib cage and extend both your arms above your head towards the ceiling.

2 Exhale, pulling your navel towards your spine and extend one arm in front of you and the other arm behind you, both at shoulder height. Feel the stretch from palm to palm. Inhale and extend your arms back above your head to your starting position. Exhale and repeat the exercise with a different arm in front each time. Repeat 10 times, maintaining the correct breathing pattern.

buttock squats

This technique tones the buttocks and thighs while increasing your circulation.

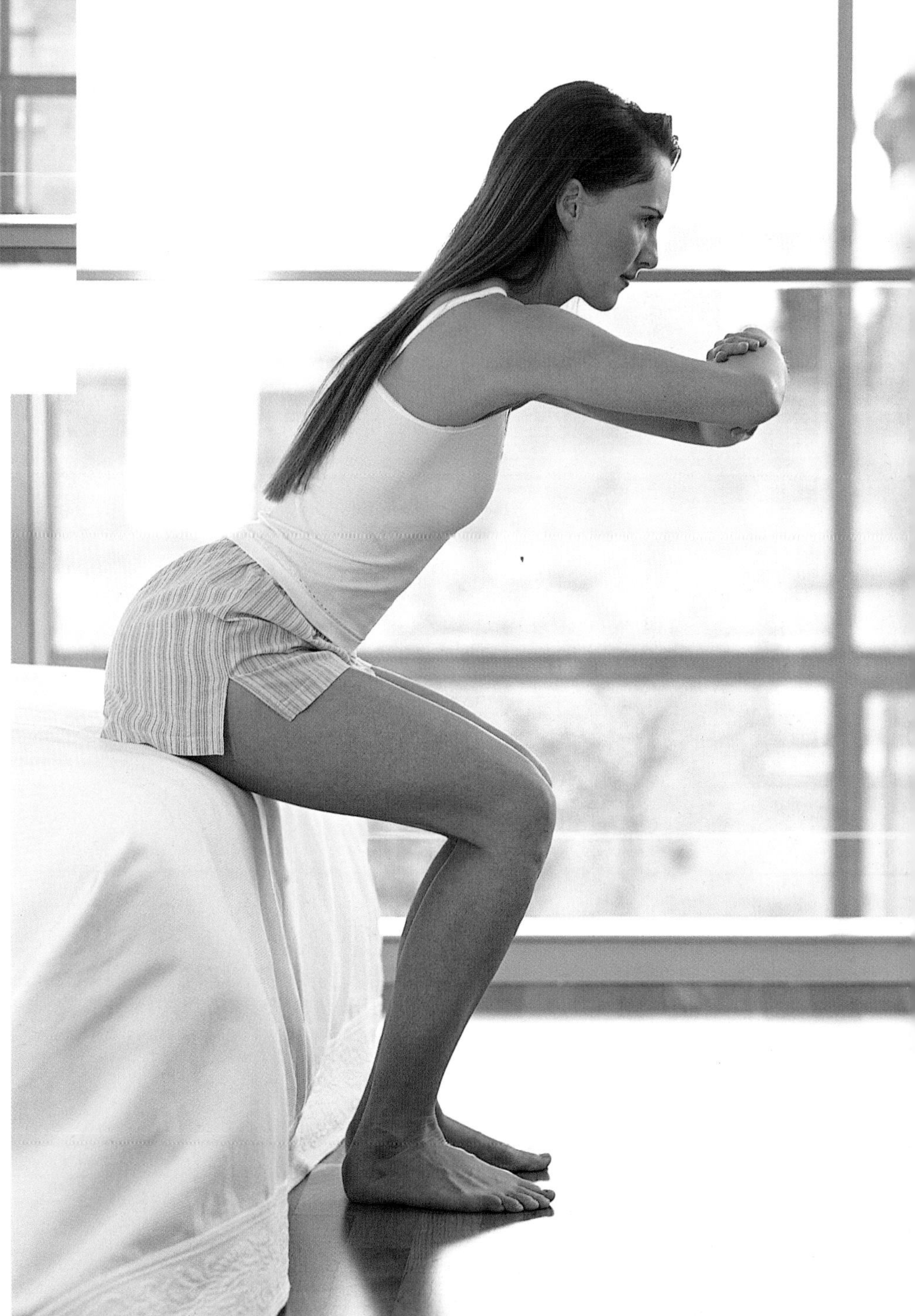

1 Stand with your back to your bed, your feet shoulder width apart and pointing forwards. Ensure your spine is erect, your abdominals engaged and your chest open. Extend your arms comfortably at chest height and place each hand on the opposite elbow. Inhale.

2 Exhale as you squat down to touch the edge of your bed lightly with your buttocks. Inhale as you stand upright again. Repeat 15 times then rest.

arm toners

A great way to get those arms pumping, this exercise tones the back of your arms and your chest muscles.

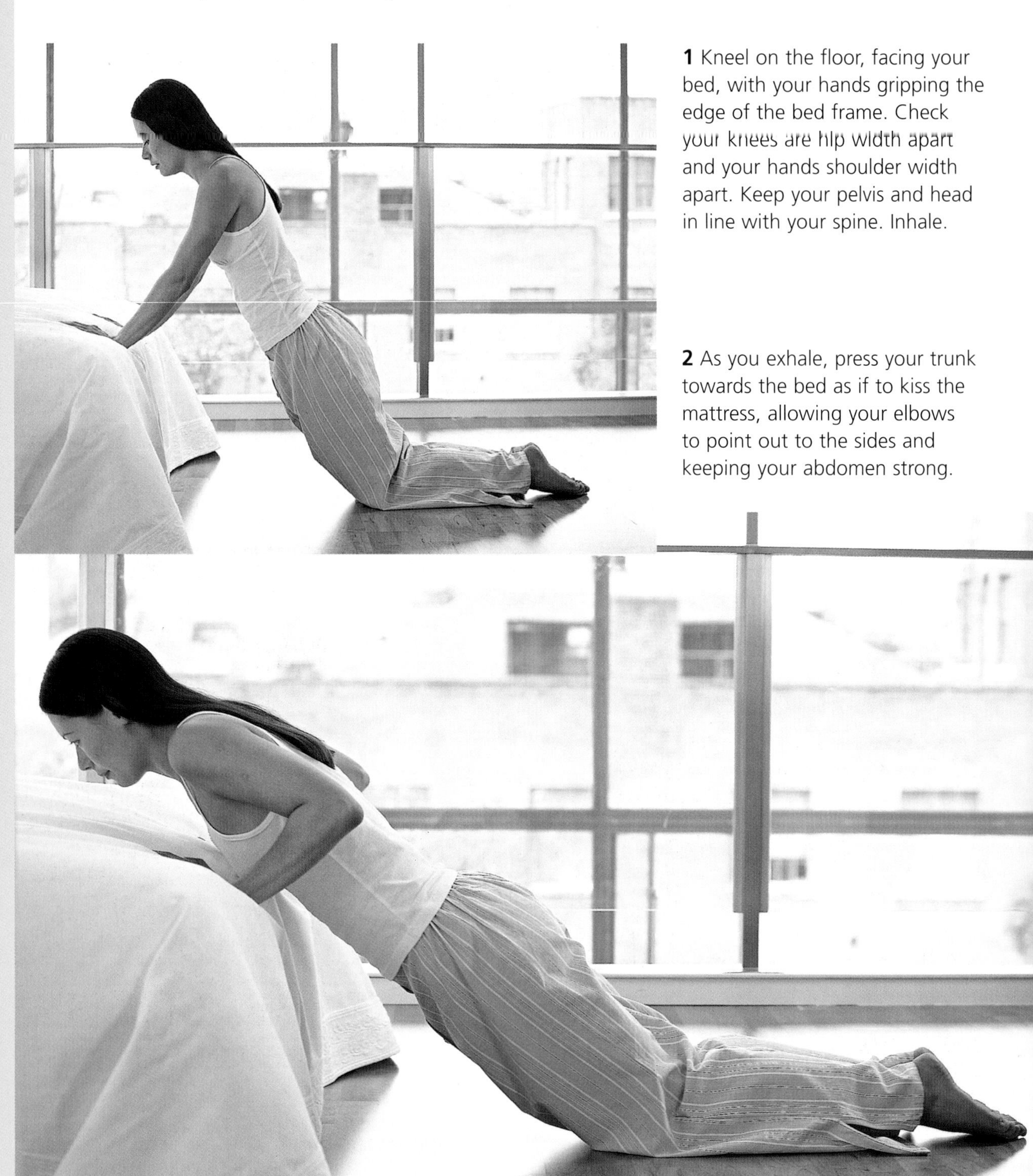

1 Kneel on the floor, facing your bed, with your hands gripping the edge of the bed frame. Check your knees are hip width apart and your hands shoulder width apart. Keep your pelvis and head in line with your spine. Inhale.

2 As you exhale, press your trunk towards the bed as if to kiss the mattress, allowing your elbows to point out to the sides and keeping your abdomen strong.

variation

1 To make the exercise more challenging, extend both legs behind you. Support your upper body on your outstretched arms and keep your legs strong so you can rest on the balls of your feet. Keep your whole body in one straight line from head to toe. Inhale.

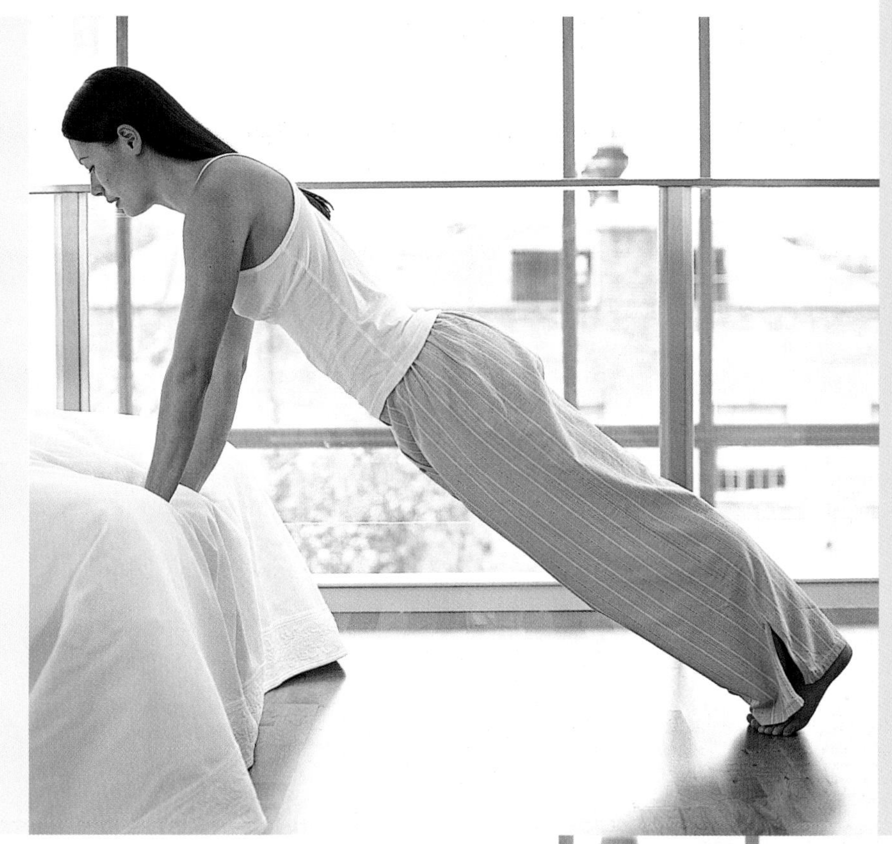

2 As you exhale, press your trunk towards the bed as before, keeping your body in a single line. Repeat 8–12 times.

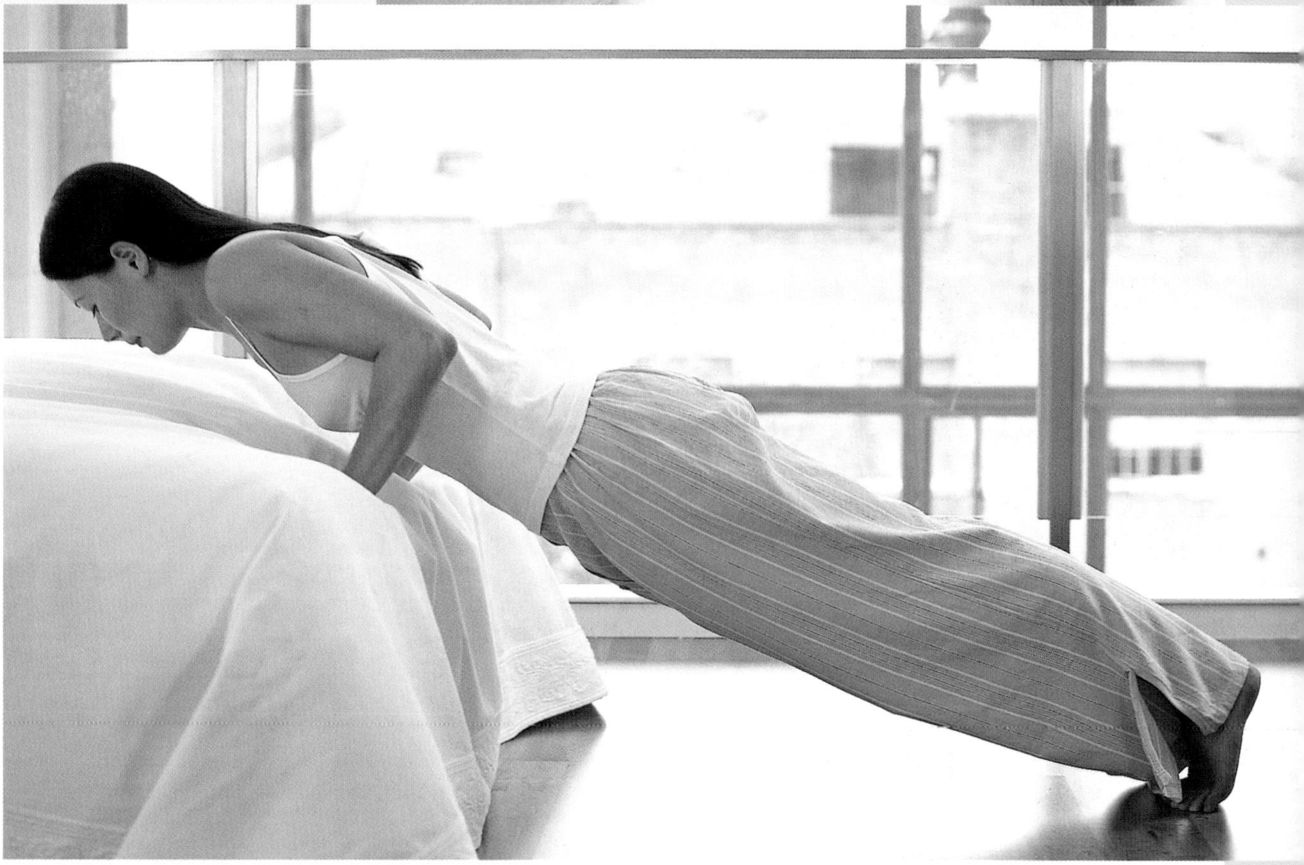

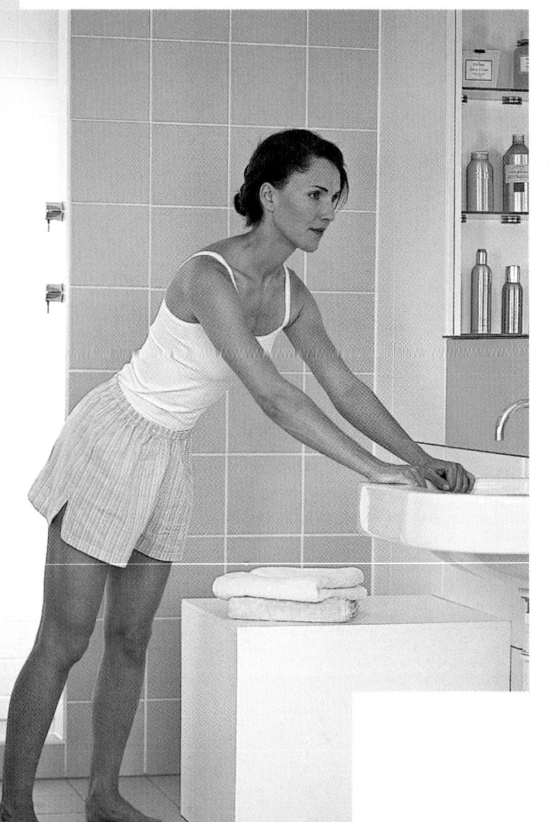

back release

This keeps your spine supple, opens your chest and brings energy and vitality.

1 Place your hands shoulder width apart on the edge of the bathroom basin. Walk backwards until your arms are straight and your legs are at right angles to your trunk. Inhale and, keeping your arms straight, bring your hips towards the basin and lift your head. Lift your heels and, keeping your legs straight, move your sacrum (tail bone) inwards. Move your shoulders down, lift your chest and, breathing out, look upwards. Hold for 3–5 slow cycles of breathing. Breathe out and return to the right-angle position.

2 Drop your head below your arms to stretch your neck. Keep your abdomen pulled in and your chest open. Hold for 5 cycles of slow breathing.

chest opener

This technique opens the chest and stretches and tones the muscles in your chest and the back of your arms.

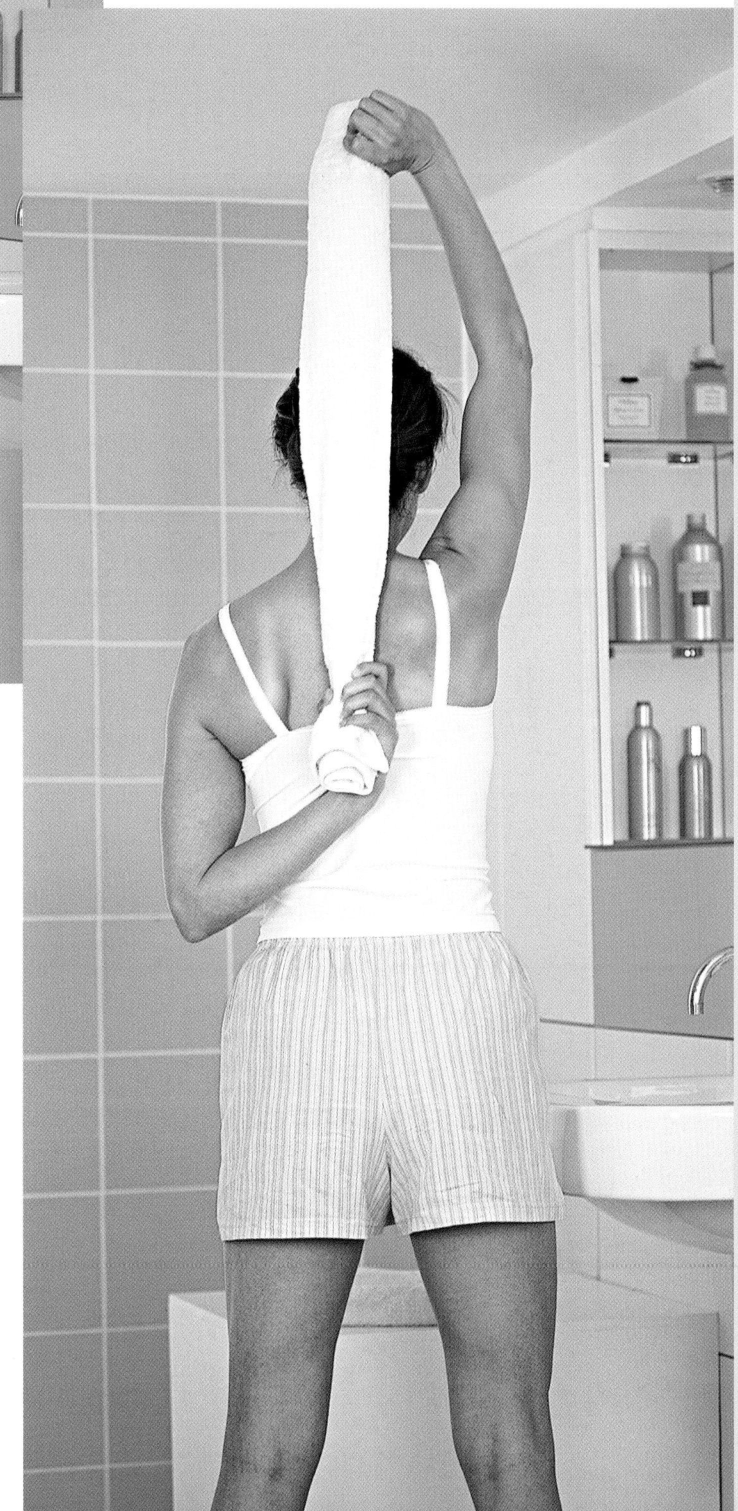

1 Stand with your feet hip width apart, ensuring your knees are slightly soft, your back elongated and your abdominal muscles engaged. Firmly grip each end of a rolled-up towel and hold it vertically behind your back.

2 Inhale as you pull the towel in an upward direction towards the ceiling. Then exhale as you pull the towel downwards in the opposite direction – as though drying your back between your shoulder blades. Repeat 20 times, breathing correctly and ensuring your shoulders remain level.

waist trimmer

Release tension in the small discs in your back that help to maintain rotational movement of the spine.

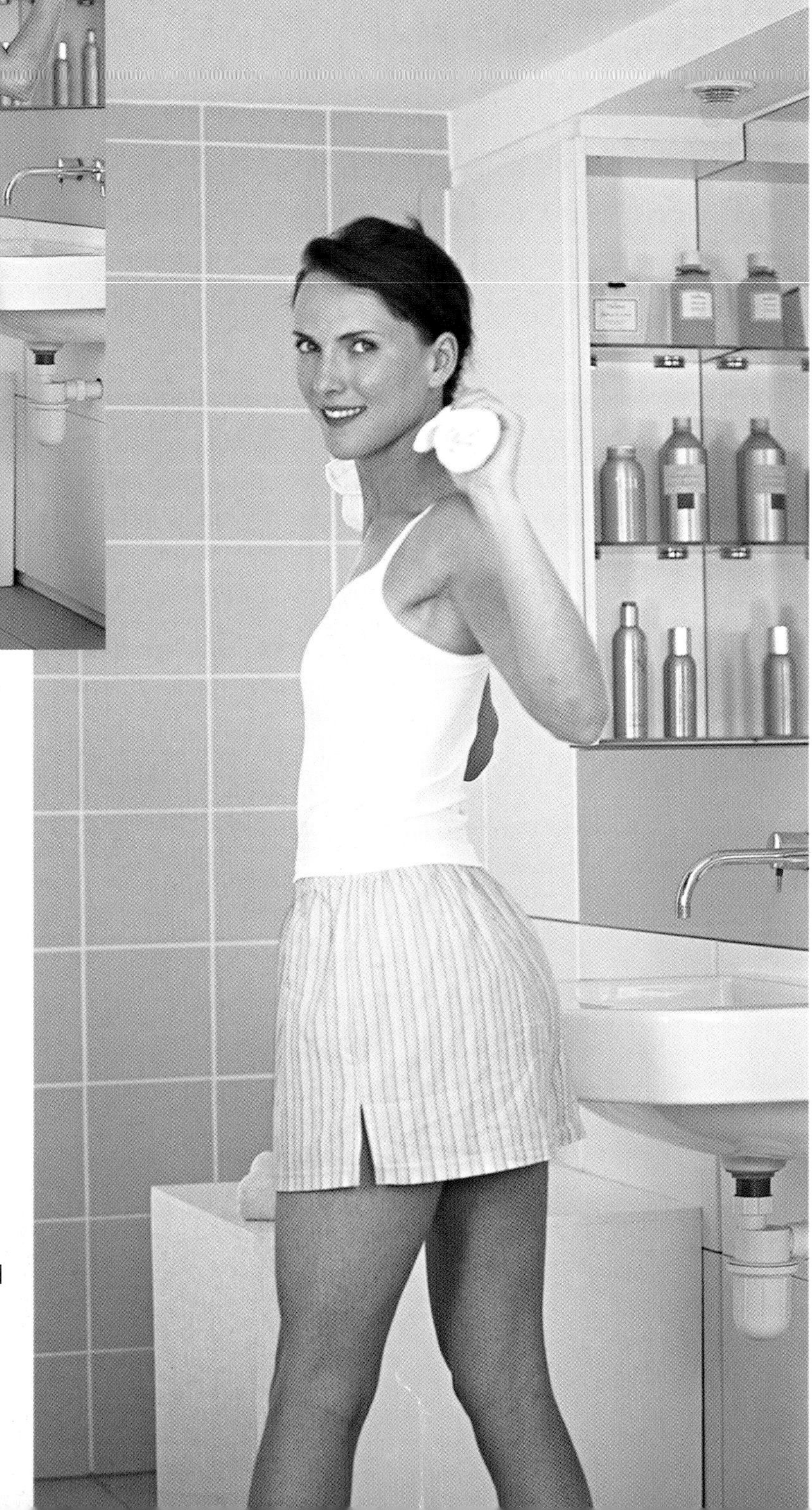

1 Stand with your feet shoulder width apart, making sure your spine is erect, your abdominal muscles engaged and your chest open. Firmly grip each end of a rolled-up towel and hold it behind your neck, taking care not to pull your head forwards.

2 Inhale fully then exhale and rotate your trunk to the right, keeping your shoulders level. Inhale as you come back to the centre position, then exhale and rotate your trunk to the left. Repeat 20 times, ensuring you breathe correctly.

shoulder strengthener

This is another exercise that uses a towel to improve shoulder strength and tones the arms.

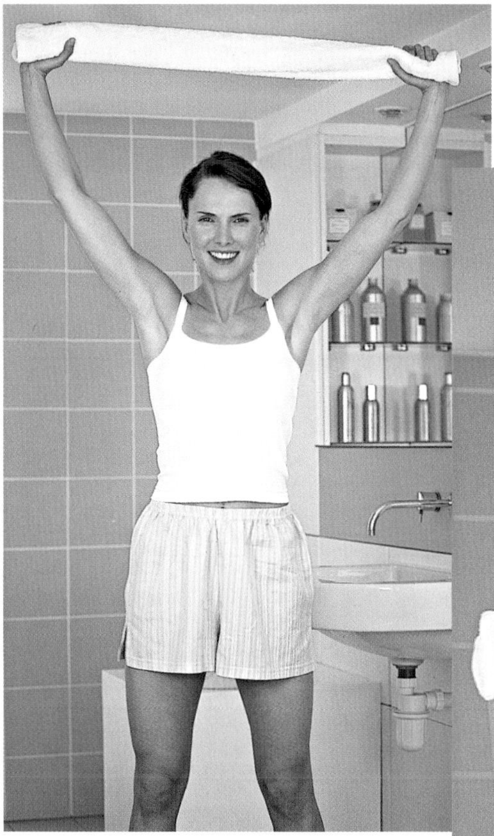

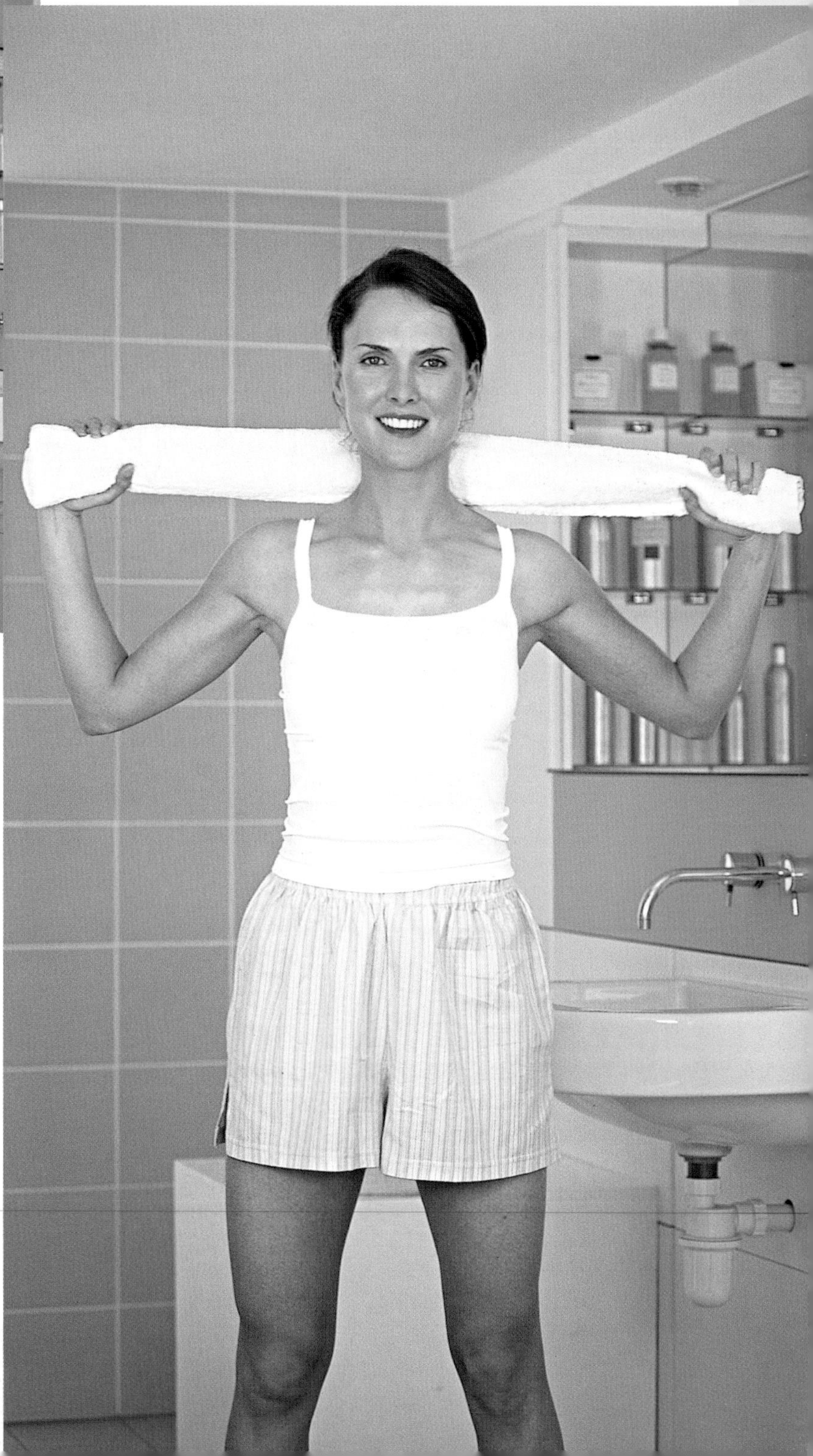

1 Stand with your feet shoulder width apart and your knees slightly soft. Firmly hold each end of a rolled-up towel in front of your neck. Inhale. As you exhale lift the towel into the air, keeping it slightly in front of your shoulders.

2 Inhale. As you exhale lower the towel behind your head without pressing your head forwards. Repeat 10 times, ensuring you breathe correctly.

right-angled basin bend

Use the washbasin to stretch your arms and shoulders, and relieve stiff legs. This exercise helps to prevent headaches.

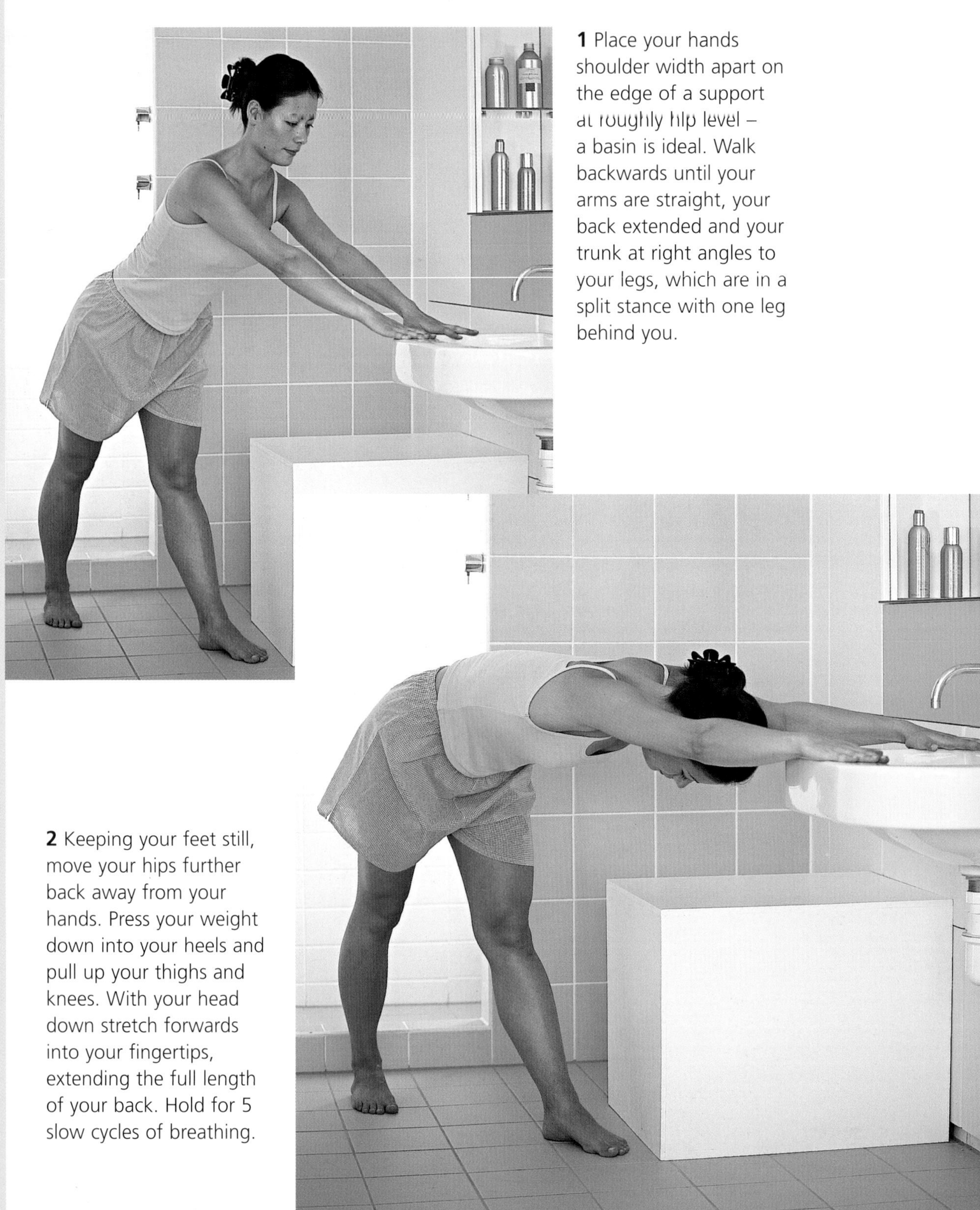

1 Place your hands shoulder width apart on the edge of a support at roughly hip level – a basin is ideal. Walk backwards until your arms are straight, your back extended and your trunk at right angles to your legs, which are in a split stance with one leg behind you.

2 Keeping your feet still, move your hips further back away from your hands. Press your weight down into your heels and pull up your thighs and knees. With your head down stretch forwards into your fingertips, extending the full length of your back. Hold for 5 slow cycles of breathing.

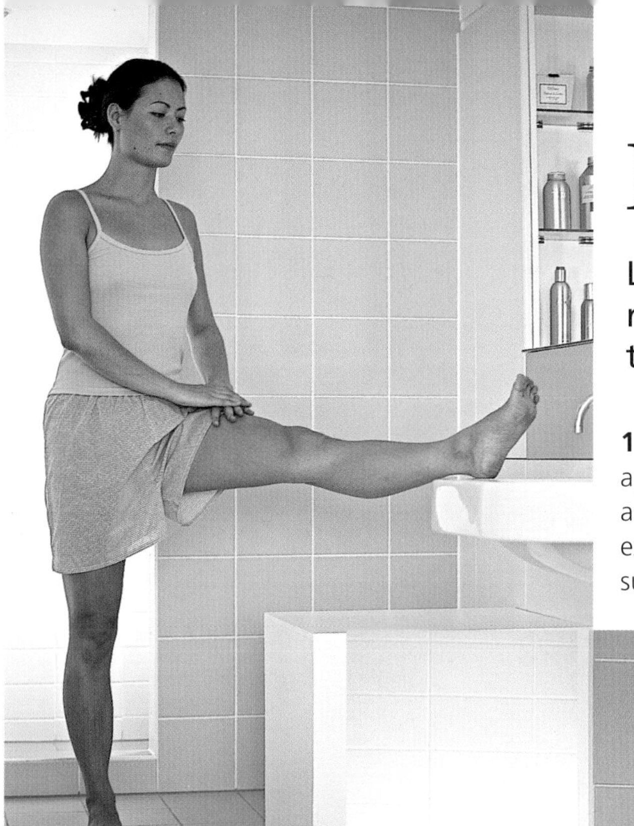

leg stretch

Lengthen your hamstrings and release the lower spine with this bathroom stretch.

1 Stand with your feet hip width apart. Check your hips are level and your feet stable. Inhale and extend your left leg up to rest on a support such as a basin.

2 Exhale and lean forwards to stretch your trunk over your left leg, while pulling the left thigh muscle into the thigh bone. Breathe in and release your trunk then exhale and stretch a little further. Hold the stretch for 1–2 minutes. Repeat the stretch with the other leg.

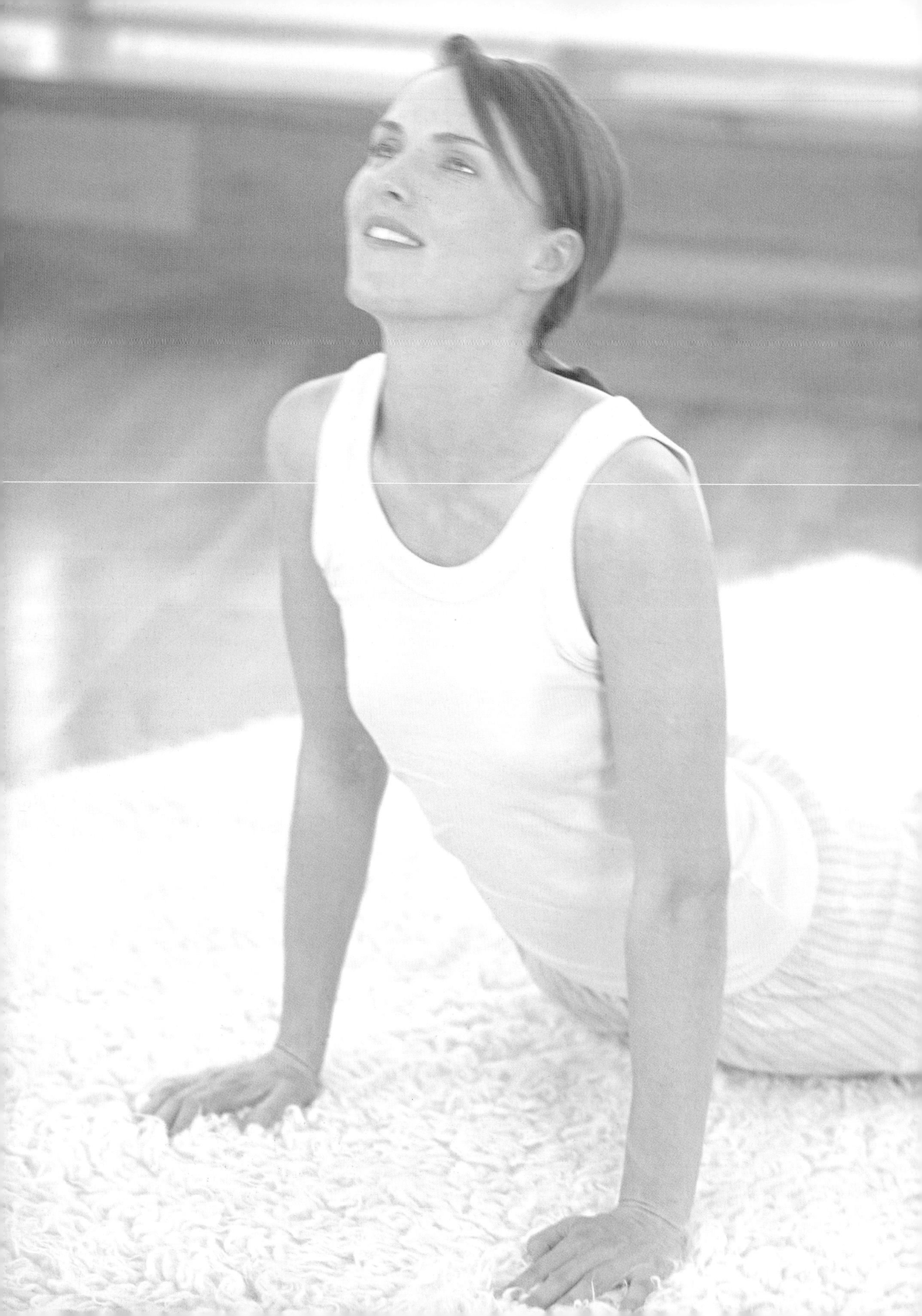

wake up with yoga

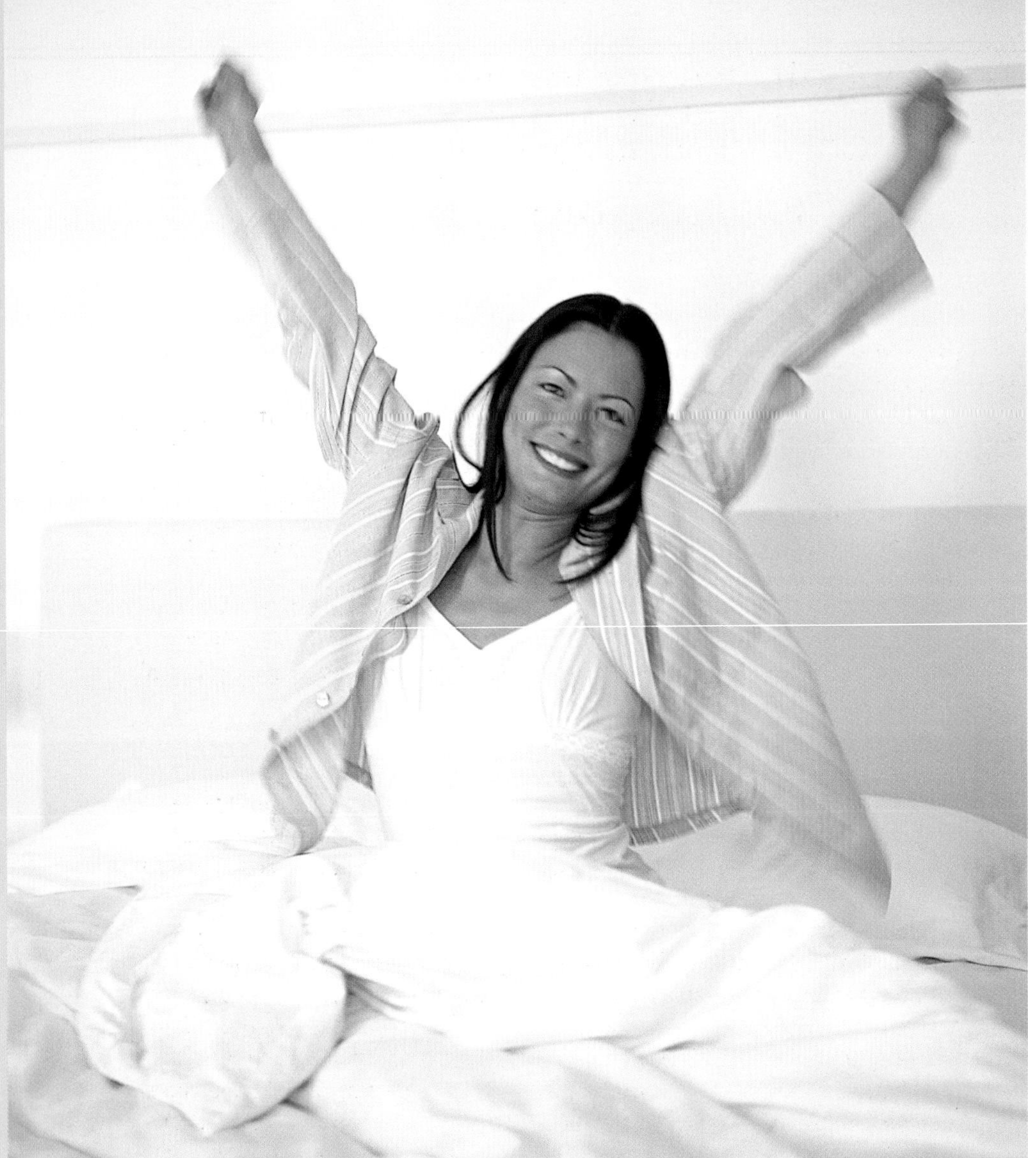

wake up with yoga

Yoga, which means union of breath and body, is an age-old mix of spiritual awareness and physical discipline, which was developed in India around 5,000 years ago. One of the six orthodox systems of Indian philosophy, it was collated and systemized by Patanjali, in his classical work, the Yoga Sutras.

Why do yoga?

Yoga will help you to relax and will tone and strengthen your muscles at the same time. It is a very subtle art of moving gently and using the breath to soften the inner body. This means that the synergy of the breath is timed exactly with the body's movement, thereby softening the interconnective tissue between muscle and bone.

Yoga first thing in the morning is one of the best things you can do for yourself. There is no better time to reap the rewards of this eastern practice and enhance your

'If you feel a bit groggy in the morning there is nothing to beat a little early morning yoga'

body's flexibility, recharge your energy, loosen your joints, centre your mind and boost your concentration.

The ullolas and vinyasas (see pages 56–57 and 58–67), traditionally performed at sunrise, are possibly the best exercise sequences in the entire universe. This is because they are fluid in nature, suitable for all levels and gently soften your body into the day, safely and effectively. A few rounds at the start of the day will completely energize you and leave you raring to go. In your 10-minute morning workout you will be able to complete 10 full vinyasas or a selection of ullolas.

Morning is also the ideal time for breathing exercises (see page 34) and meditation. Breathing exercises make you more aware of your breath, and breathing properly is a technique that needs to be practised. Breathing practice enhances your capacity to stay calm, open and relaxed in stressful times.

Any time of day

If you do miss your morning session, yoga is a good routine to perform when you get home from work in the evening. It will release your mind from the day's events and free any tension in your body. It will also help you get a good night's sleep in preparation for the next day's wake-up workout.

The body is commonly tighter in the mornings – after a night spent sleeping in a horizontal position, which creates tension in your spine, neck and legs – and you may feel that you cannot perform some of the yoga postures as well as you can in the evening. Do not be concerned – it simply means that your body takes longer to soften in the morning than it does in the evening. You are more sensitive in the morning and also more aware of your breathing since it is easier to focus mentally at this time before the distractions of the day start. Once this awareness of your breathing deepens with practise, you will be able to trace build-ups of stress or tension in your breathing at work or in stressful situations and you will be able to deal with them quicker.

BE FLEXIBLE

If you intend to perform any evening workouts, make sure you do so within 30 minutes of getting home. Otherwise you will be distracted by the hundreds of things that always need to be done. And, as soon as you hit the sofa – let's be honest – you'll forget all about working out!

ullolas

This breathing preparation sequence is designed to soften your spine and pelvis before starting the vinyasa sequence on pages 58–59.

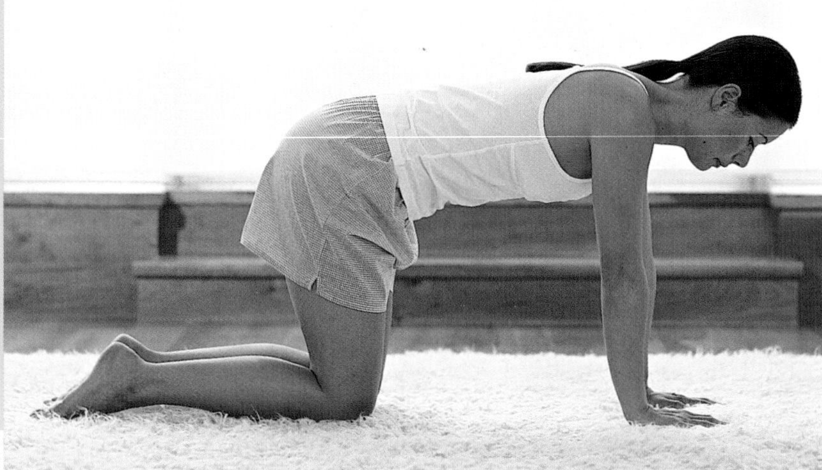

1 Kneel on all fours with your hands flat on the floor directly beneath your shoulders and your hips directly above your knees. Spread your fingers on the floor to take your weight evenly.

2 Inhale through your nose and as you exhale bend your elbows and lower your trunk towards the floor – but don't touch it. Ensure your weight is evenly distributed over your right and left hands and your elbows are behind your wrists.

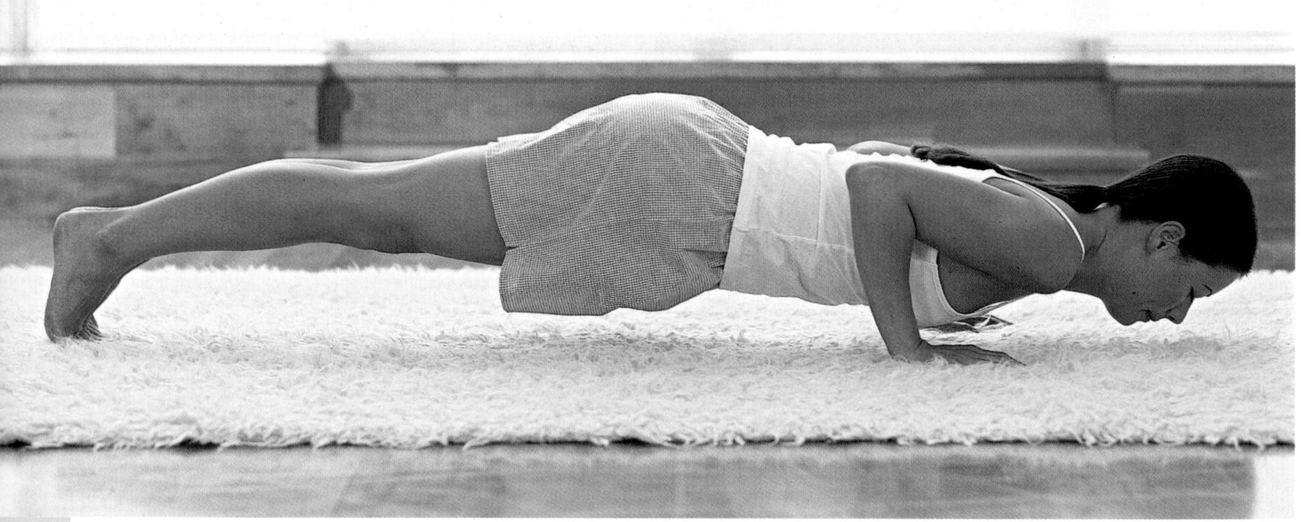

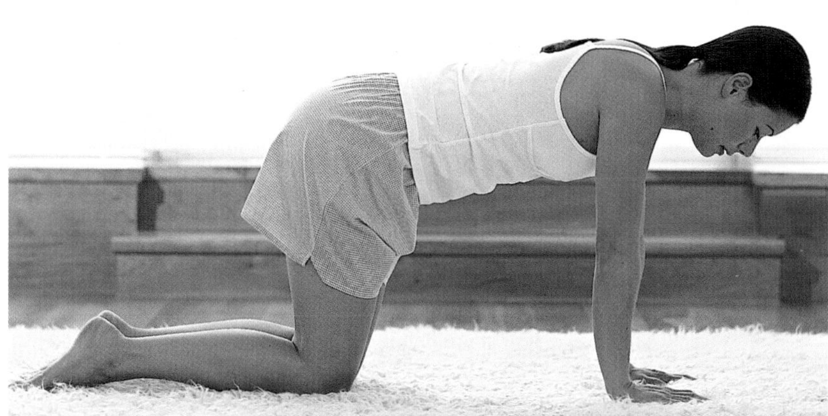

3 Inhale and return to your starting position.

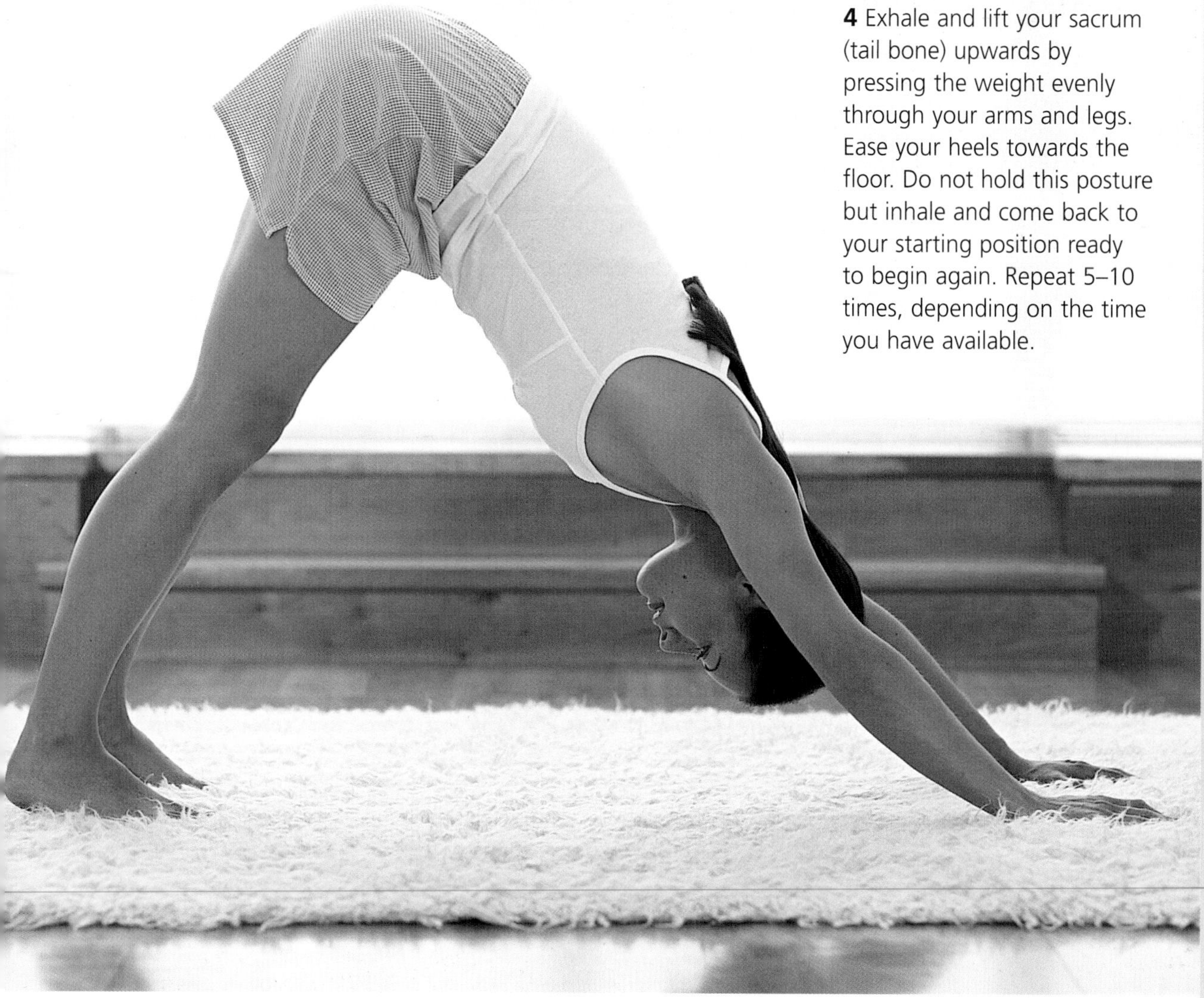

4 Exhale and lift your sacrum (tail bone) upwards by pressing the weight evenly through your arms and legs. Ease your heels towards the floor. Do not hold this posture but inhale and come back to your starting position ready to begin again. Repeat 5–10 times, depending on the time you have available.

vinyasas

More intense than the ullolas, the vinyasas increase circulation, muscular strength and flexibility. The breath instructions must be adhered to.

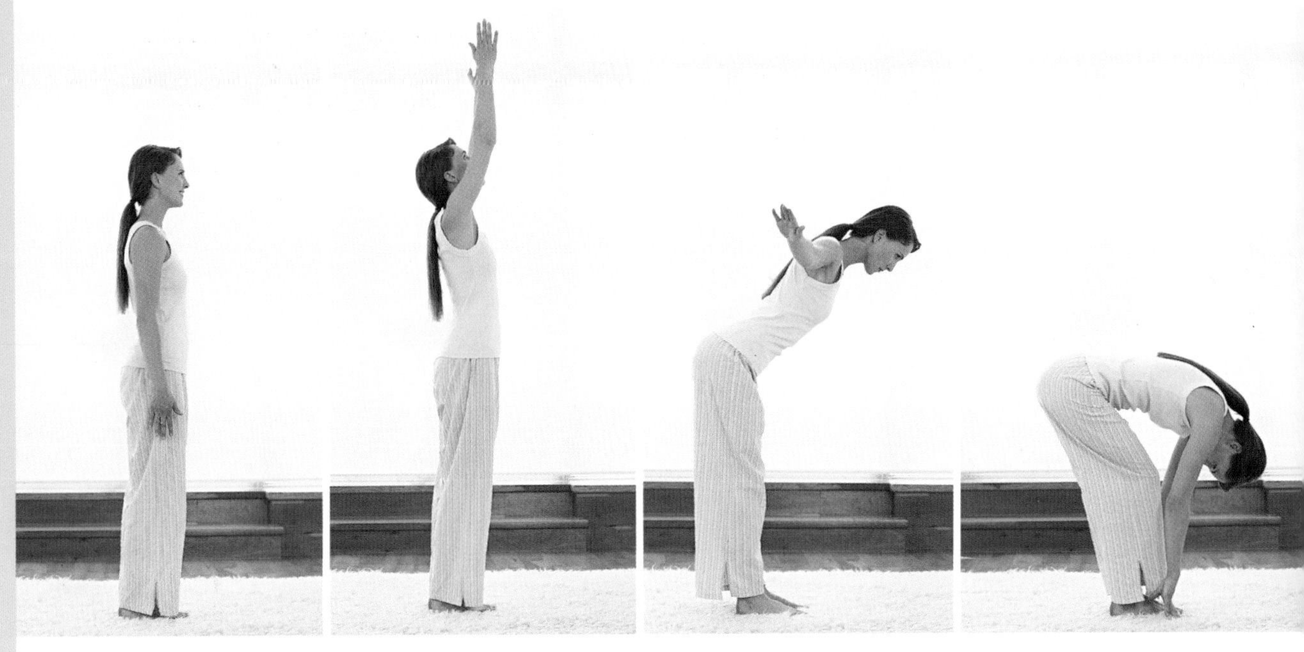

standing neutral ▶ mountain pose ▶ transition to standing fold ▶ standing fold ▶

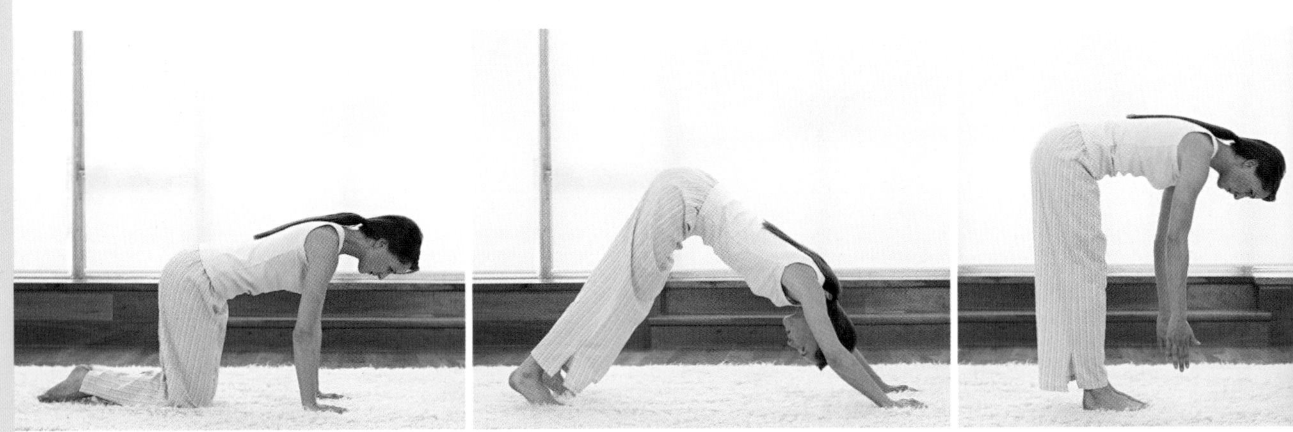

box position ▶ downward-facing dog ▶ active back extension ▶

These pictures show how the vinyasa progresses from movement to movement very easily. Once you have performed the sequence a few times you will soon know it without having to refer to these pages.

Go through the individual techniques (see pages 60–67) one by one when you have looked at this sequence. Note that vinyasas should be nourishing to the body and gentle. Each time you practise, refine the techniques. Do not be tempted to speed up unnaturally away from your natural breath. The breath will tell you everything, you just have to be sensitive to it and act accordingly. Repeat the whole sequence 4–12 times.

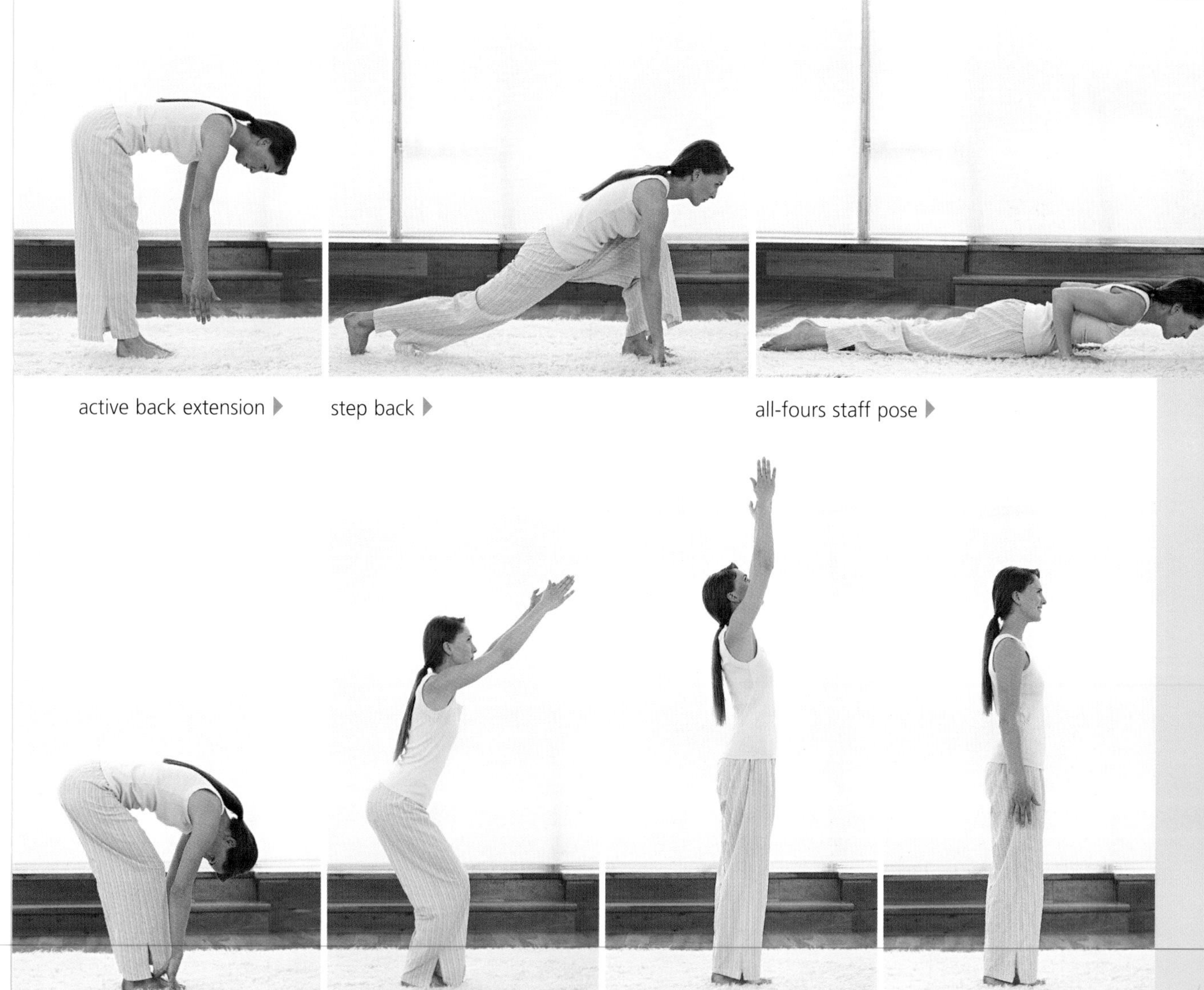

active back extension ▸ step back ▸ all-fours staff pose ▸

standing fold ▸ chair ▸ mountain pose ▸ standing neutral

active back extension

This movement opens the rib cage and strengthens shoulder retraction and abdominal/spine synergy.

1 Lengthen your trunk, breathe in deeply to expand your rib cage and open your chest. Suck your solar plexus (the stomach area beneath the diaphragm) in and up, keeping your chest active, open and full. Feel your long, soft abdomen as your sacrum (tail bone) and perineum are lifted. Inhale and keep your gaze downward, checking that your abdomen is flat and that your rib cage is full as you lengthen your spine and lift and open your chest. Rest on your fingertips if it helps to keep your spine long.

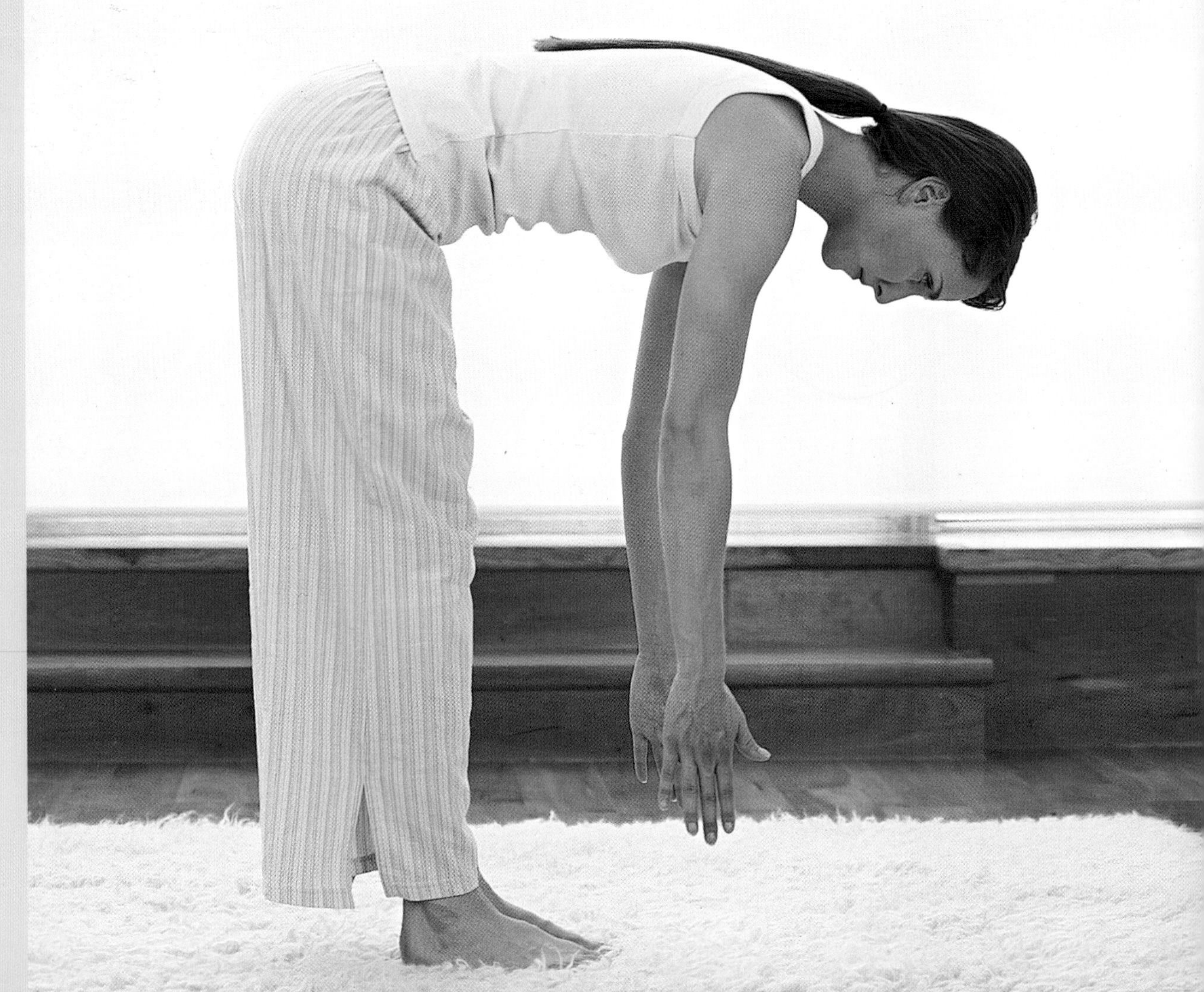

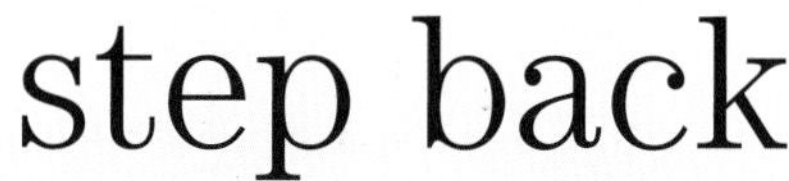

step back

Push off from hands flat on the floor to lift your legs and jump back for this movement.

1 Exhale and place your palms flat on the floor, pressing your weight evenly into every finger base on your hands. Inhale as you take your weight forwards and use your arms to step back on to the ball of each foot in turn.

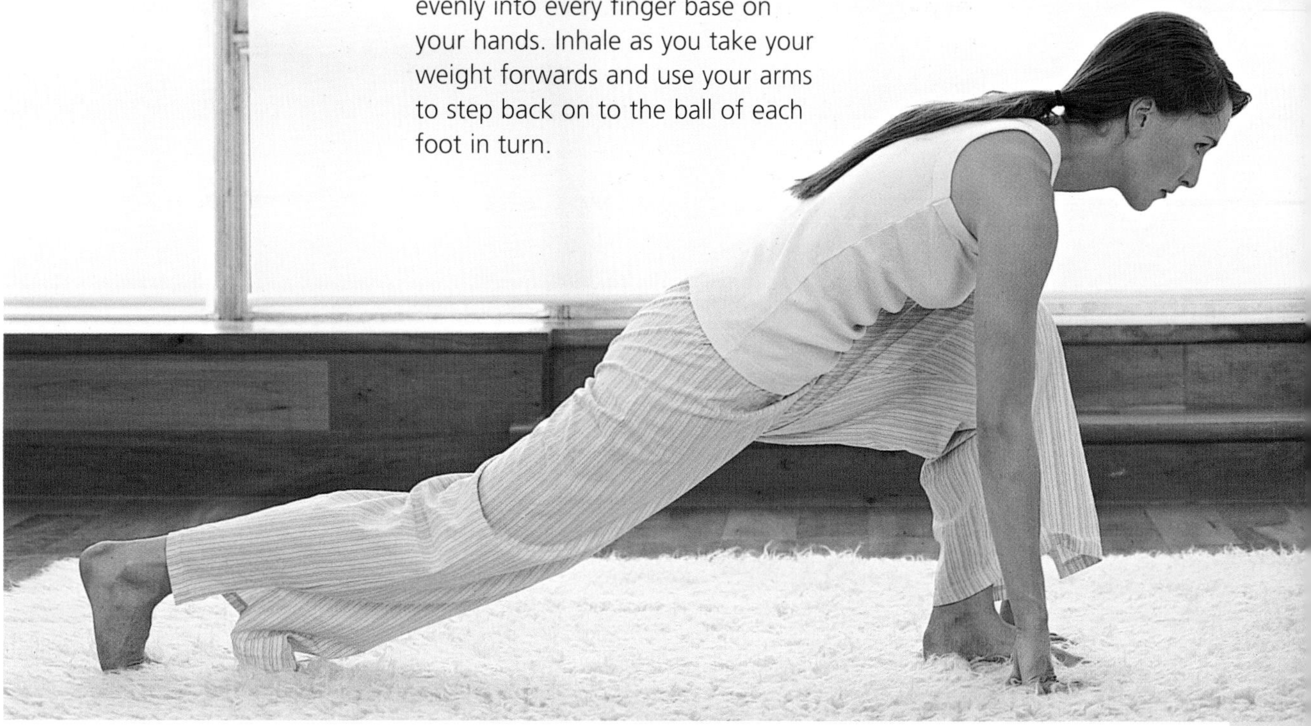

variation

Jumping back is a more advanced option – although you are definitely advised to simply step back if you have knee problems. Start as above then inhale as you take your weight forwards and push from your arms and shoulders as you lift your body up and forwards to take your legs back. Land, with your elbows bent, into the 'All-fours staff pose' (see page 64).

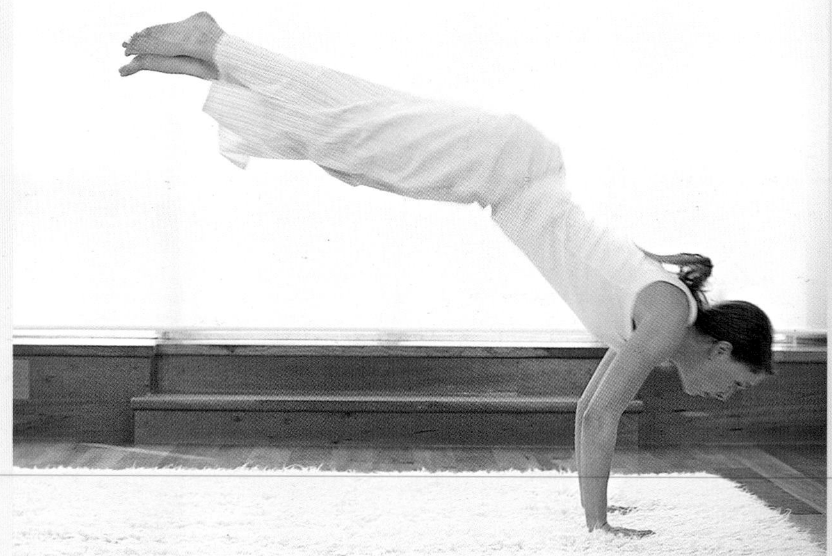

all-fours staff pose

This movement strengthens the chest, arms and triceps muscles.

1 Continuing on the same exhalation as the 'Step back' (see page 63), bend your elbows, keeping your upper arms parallel to the floor and your back extended, and bring your chin to within a few centimetres (an inch) of the floor. Bend your knees, rest your chest on the floor and look at your nose. Press your weight evenly on to your feet by pulling your thigh muscles into your thigh bones to fully engage the legs. Your hands should be in full contact with the floor – your palms broad, your fingers long and your index finger base pressing downwards.

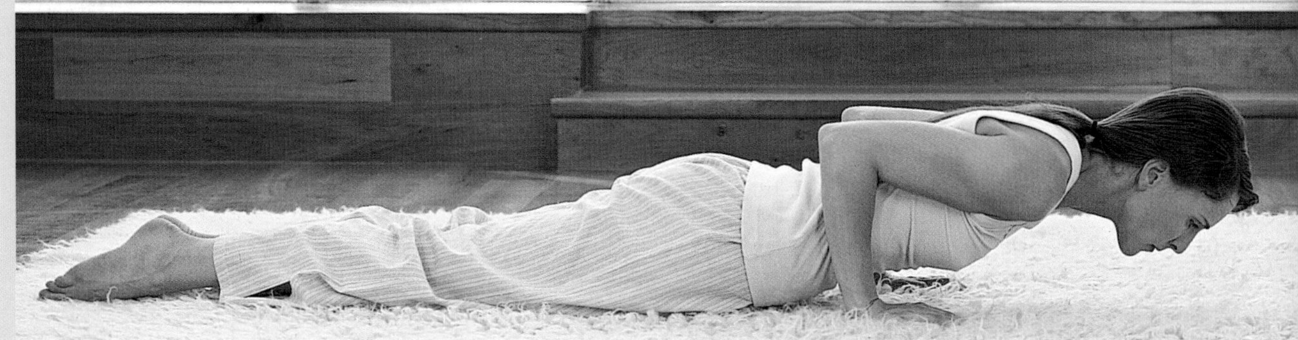

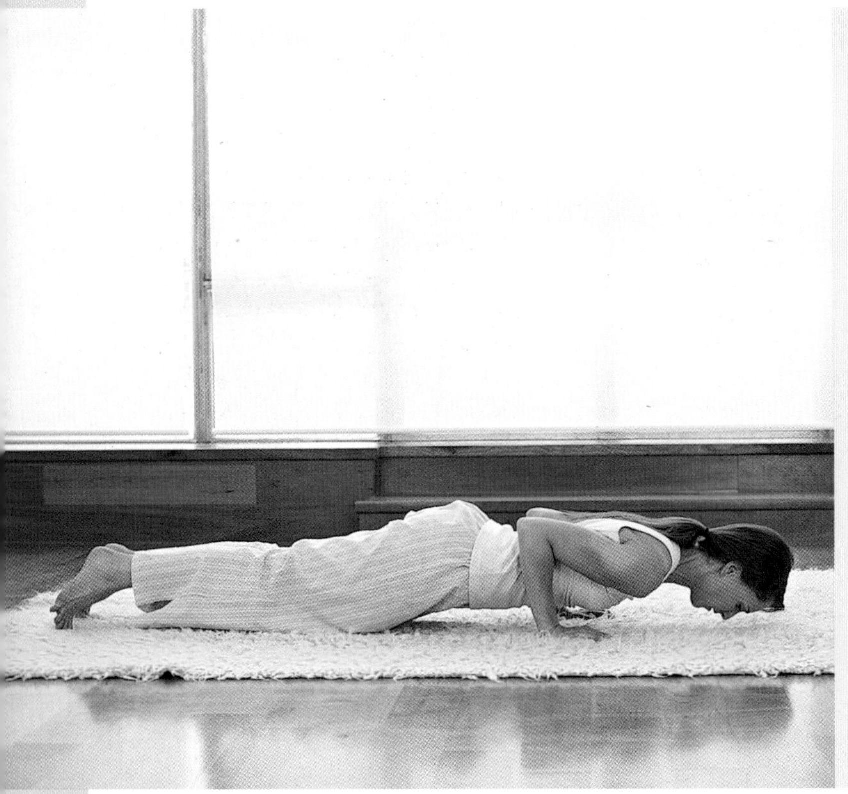

variation

This more advanced option holds the hover rather than allowing you to bend your knees and rest your chest on the floor. Continuing on the same exhalation as the 'Jump back' (see page 63), bend your elbows, keeping your upper arms parallel to the floor and your back extended, and bring your chin to within a few centimetres (an inch) of the floor. Keep your chest, pelvis and knees off the floor and look at your nose. Press your weight evenly on to both feet by pulling your thigh muscles into your thigh bones to fully engage the legs. Your hands should be in full contact with the floor – your palms broad, your fingers long and your index finger base pressing downwards.

box position

Rejuvenate your spine and strengthen your shoulders and arms with this pose.

1 Inhale and come up into a position on all fours. Practise this move until your understanding of your breathing refines. After a while you can progress from this position to practise the 'Upward-facing dog' with your knees on the floor. However, be careful that your pelvis doesn't collapse and that you have built up enough upper body strength from practising the 'All-fours staff pose' (see page 64).

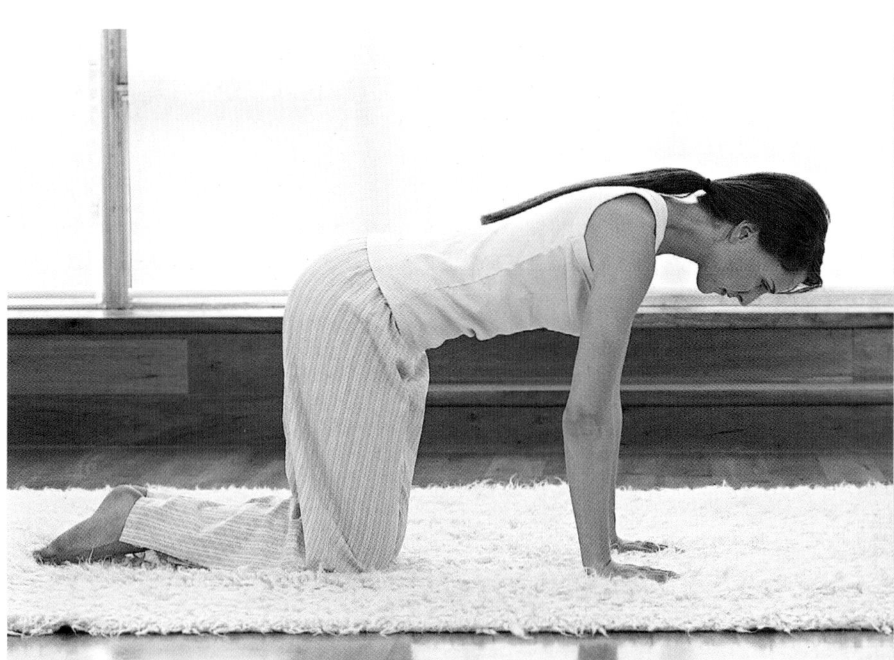

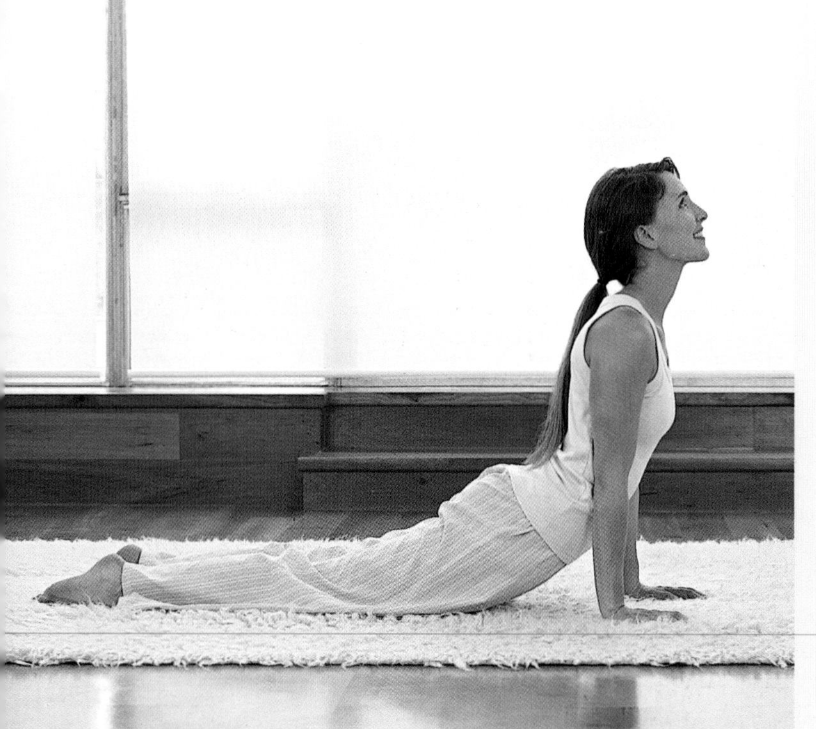

variation

Upward-facing dog is a more advanced option. Inhale as you push your chest forwards from the 'All-fours staff pose', straighten your arms and, keeping your feet where they are, roll over your toes (ensure your toenails are short!) into the 'Upward-facing dog' pose. You may need to take your hips back first to give you a little momentum to press forward through the arms and chest and roll on your toes. Spread out all your fingers to take your bodyweight and stabilize and strengthen your arms. Make sure that your knees and hips are off the floor.

downward-facing dog

This position aids digestion, lengthens your legs and spine and refines the use of your hands and feet.

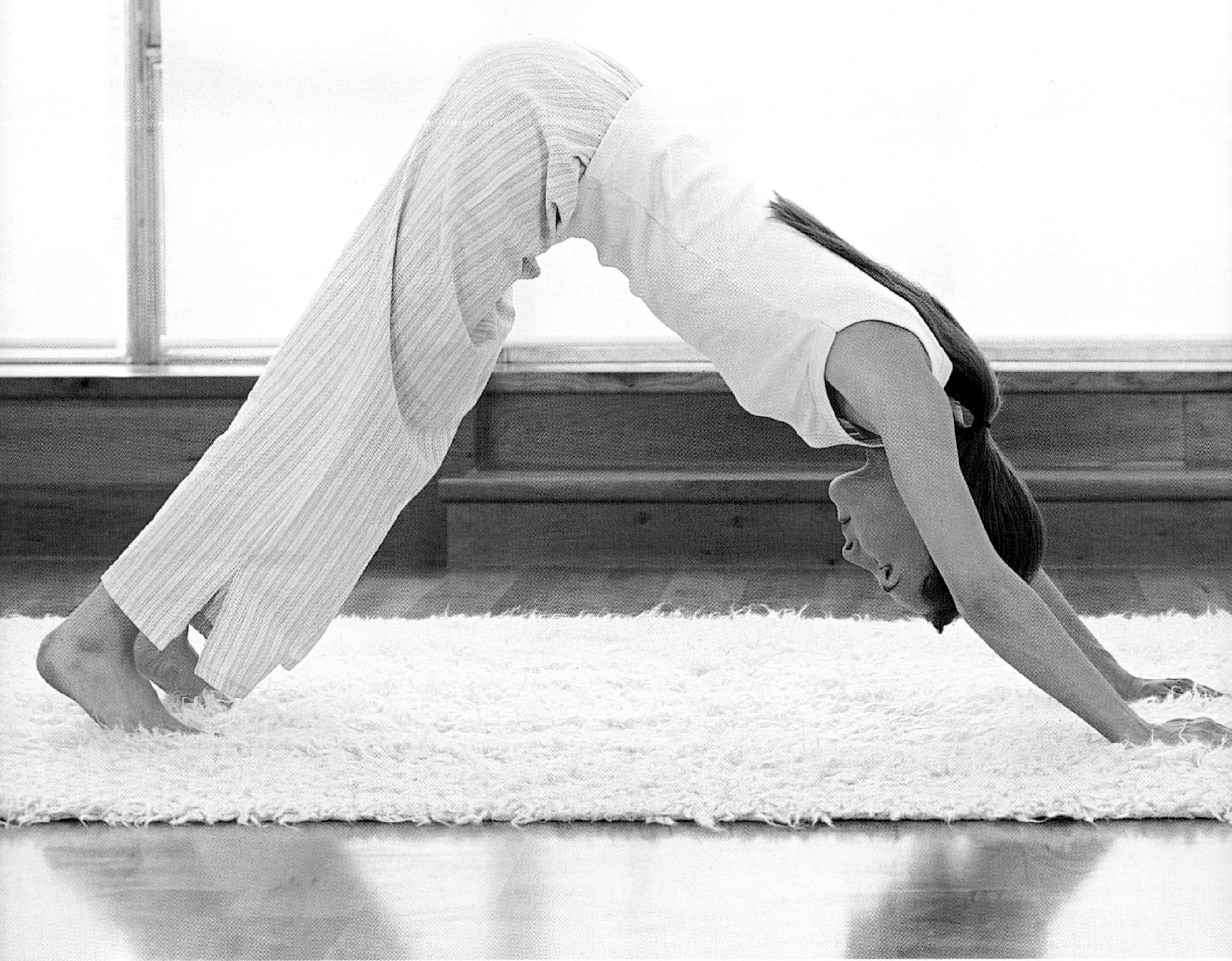

1 From the Box position (see page 65), exhale as you push up your buttocks, rolling over your toes into the 'Downward-facing dog'. Relax your head and neck totally. Keep your hands shoulder width apart, and your feet hip width apart. Your back should be extended, your arms and legs straight and your shoulders broad. Breathe deeply into your front and sides and hollow your abdomen. Do not hold the position for longer than is comfortable until your body is warmer and has softened. Rather than have straight legs, bend your knees if you feel more comfortable until your body softens and the hamstrings begin to release. Be patient and sensitive to your body's abilities.

chair

Practise this movement to strengthen your buttocks and thighs and increase your ability to balance.

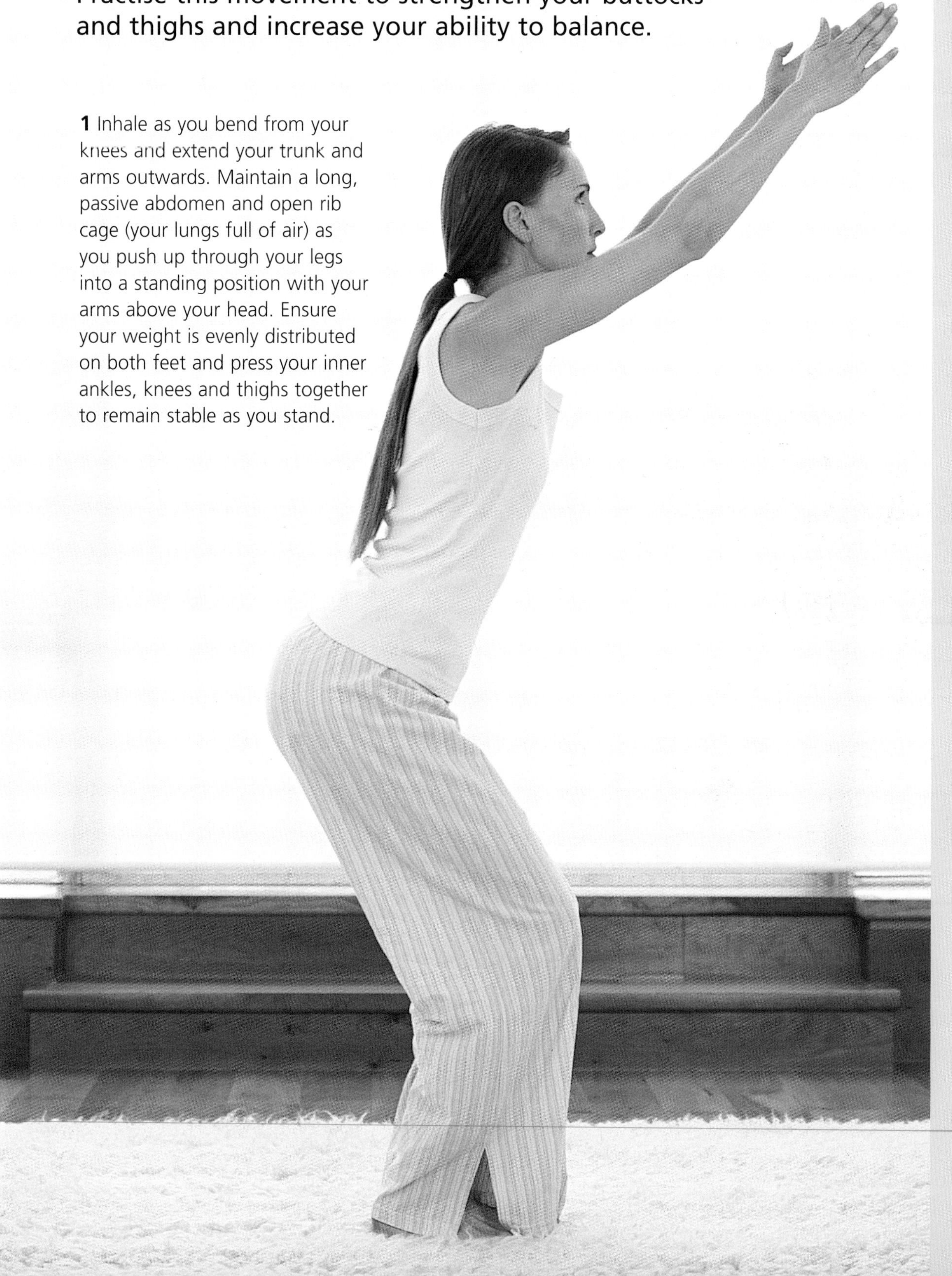

1 Inhale as you bend from your knees and extend your trunk and arms outwards. Maintain a long, passive abdomen and open rib cage (your lungs full of air) as you push up through your legs into a standing position with your arms above your head. Ensure your weight is evenly distributed on both feet and press your inner ankles, knees and thighs together to remain stable as you stand.

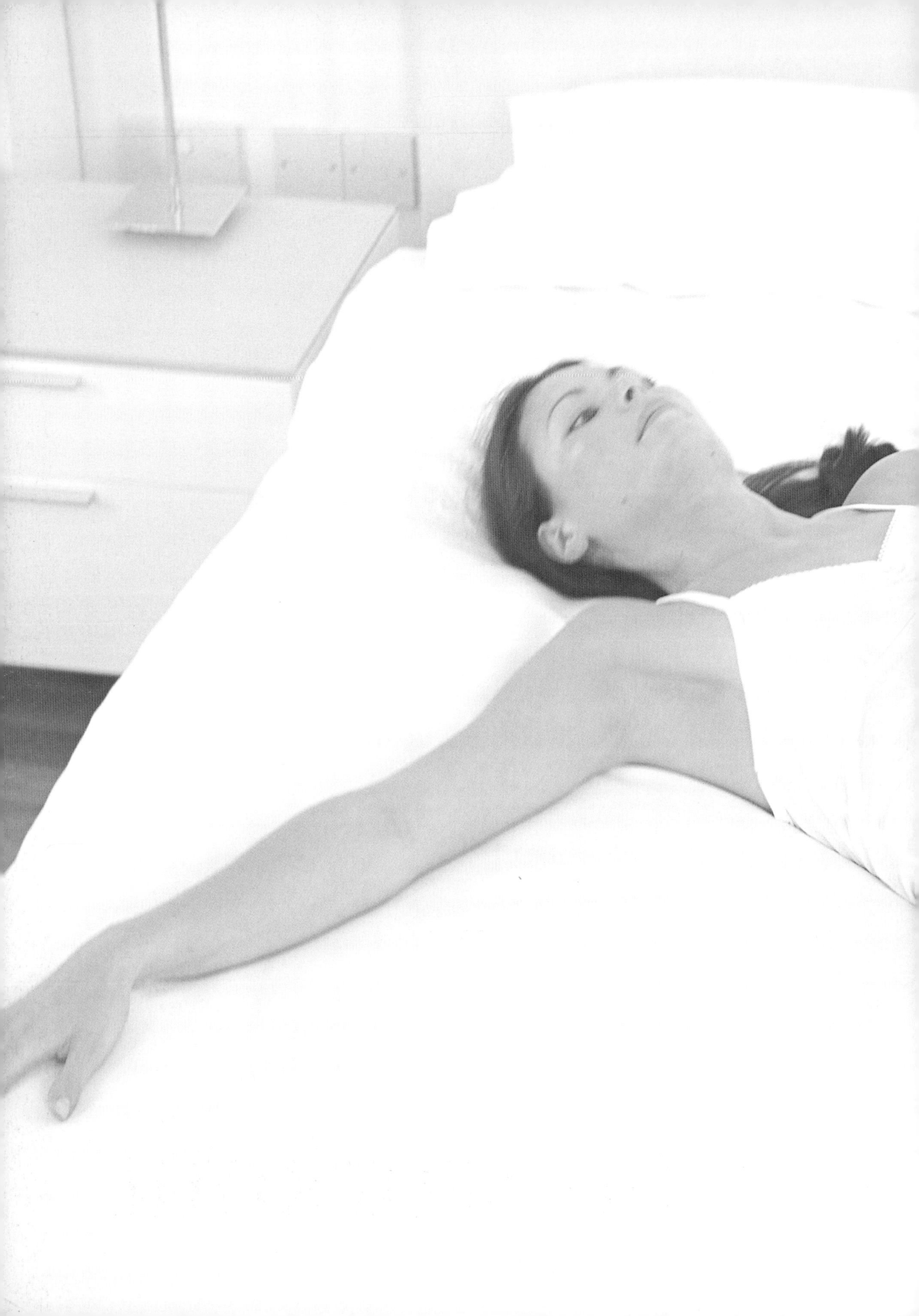

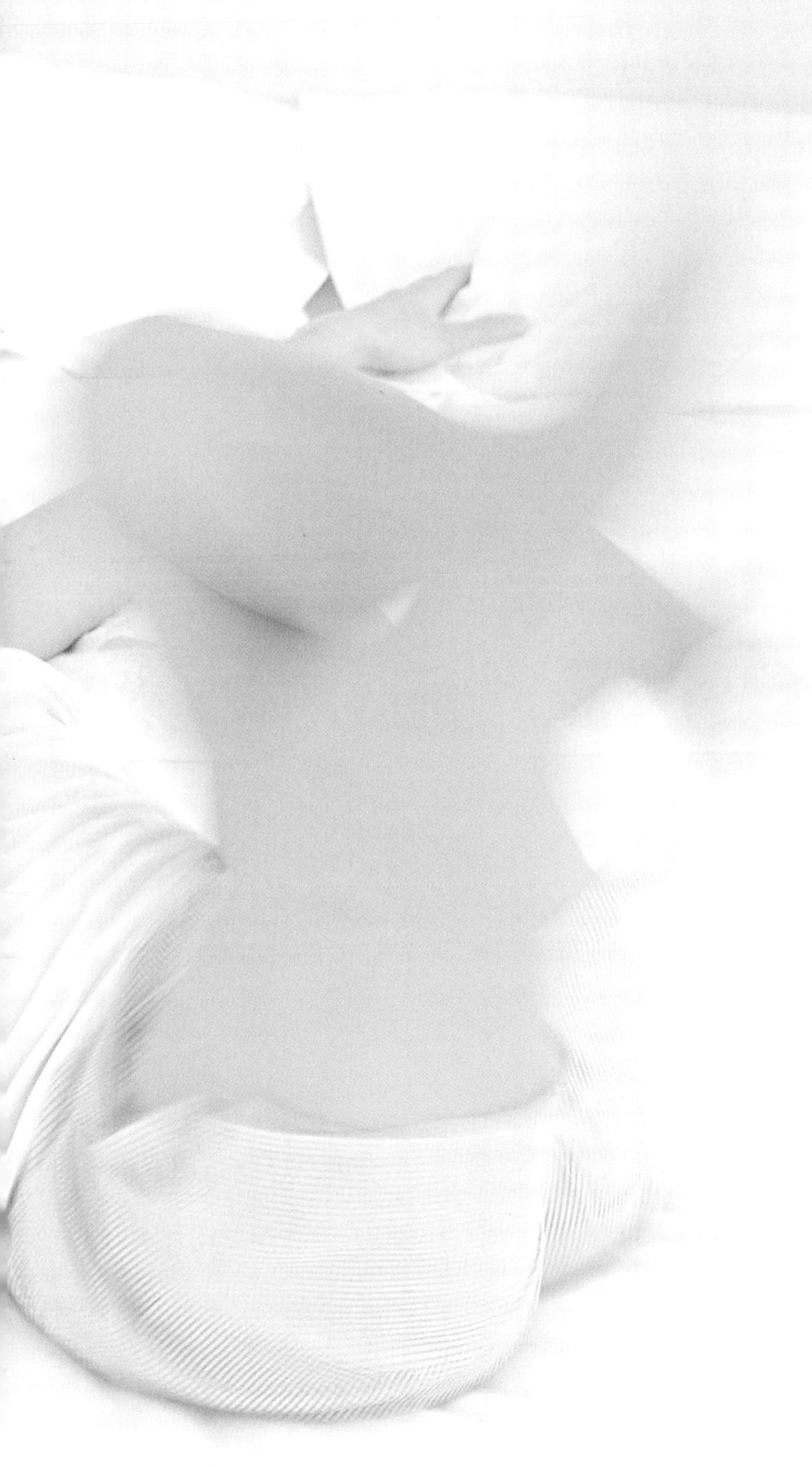

cardio workout

cardio workout

The heart is the most important muscle in the body and regular cardiovascular exercise (also known as aerobic, or fat-burning, exercise) keeps both the heart and the lungs healthy and active. According to the guidelines for improving cardiovascular fitness and body fat index issued by the American College of Sports Medicine (ACSM), cardiovascular activity should involve the large muscle groups – good examples of these activities are walking, running, cycling, stair climbing and swimming. The ACSM also recommends that you include muscular strength and flexibility training in your exercise programme, all of which have been incorporated into the 10-minute wake-up workouts.

Heart health

There are millions of deaths worldwide every year from heart-related illnesses, yet authorities like the British Heart Foundation believe the majority of coronary heart disease is potentially preventable. Prevention involves leading a normal active lifestyle with a well-balanced diet, no smoking and moderate but frequent bouts of exercise in accordance with the ACSM guidelines for health and exercise (see page 6).

BENEFITS OF ALL-ROUND EXERCISE

Combining cardiovascular exercise with the other elements of the 10-minute wake-up workouts has the following benefits:

- Lowers blood pressure and heart rate
- Burns fat
- Increases blood supply to all areas of the body
- Improves muscle tone
- Increases the resistance to fatigue
- Enhances general appearance
- Improves ability to relax

Breaking your fast

The word breakfast is made up of the words 'break' and 'fast', and the meal is just that since you effectively fast when you sleep at night. You should have your breakfast within the first few hours of rising otherwise your sugar levels will crash to an uncomfortable low.

Once you've completed your 10-minute wake-up workout routine it is time to nourish your digestive system. You need an energy-boosting breakfast that is good for

'Regular cardiovascular exercise keeps your heart and lungs healthy'

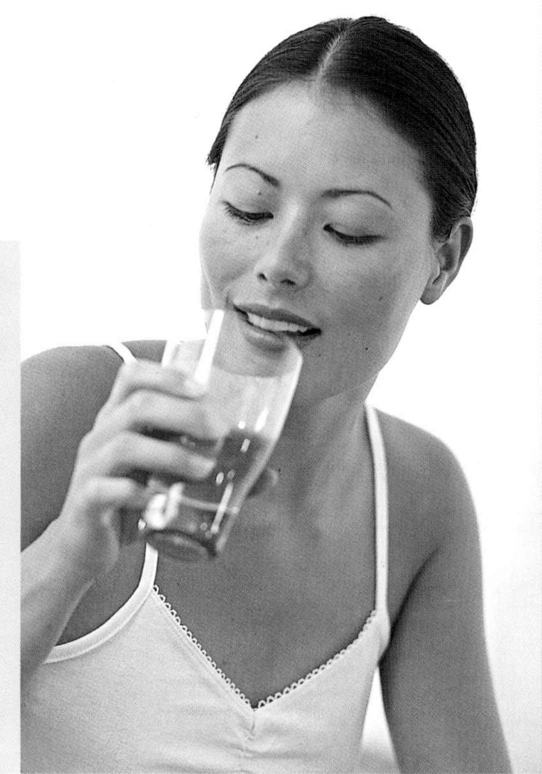

ENERGY-BOOSTING SMOOTHIE

For a very rich, extremely thick smoothie that gives you a boost for the day, juice 6 ripe pears and 2 large oranges, then pour into a blender. Add 2 stoned apricots, ½ banana, a small pinch of ground cinnamon and 6 mint leaves. Blend for 45 seconds then serve.

the heart and will keep you going all morning. Exercise can actually decrease cravings and you are more likely to eat a sensible breakfast after your workout than if you didn't exercise.

Healthy breakfast options

Many breakfast cereals are refined carbohydrates offering empty calories and minimal goodness, so a wholegrain cereal with a low fat content is the best choice. If you can't forgo your favourite cereal first thing, add fruit to it, especially pineapple, blueberries, raspberries or prunes for a really healthy breakfast.

Smoothies and juices are a good breakfast option and the quickest and most effective way of getting nutrients into your system. You will need a blender and possibly a juicer if you intend making them regularly (see box above).

Avoid heavily processed foods. Some bread fits this category, a food that many of us load our bodies with first thing in the morning. Try to select stone-ground wheat bread and avoid white bread completely. Stone grinding is one of the best ways to make bread while retaining the nutrients. Look for natural products or those with the least number of additives or preservatives.

Water

Make it your habit to drink lots of water – preferably eight glasses – throughout the day. Water flushes waste chemicals from your body and helps all your internal organs to work more efficiently. If your urine is not clear in colour then you are dehydrated. Some people spend their whole lives dehydrated, which has a negative effect on their skin, toxin removal and liver activity.

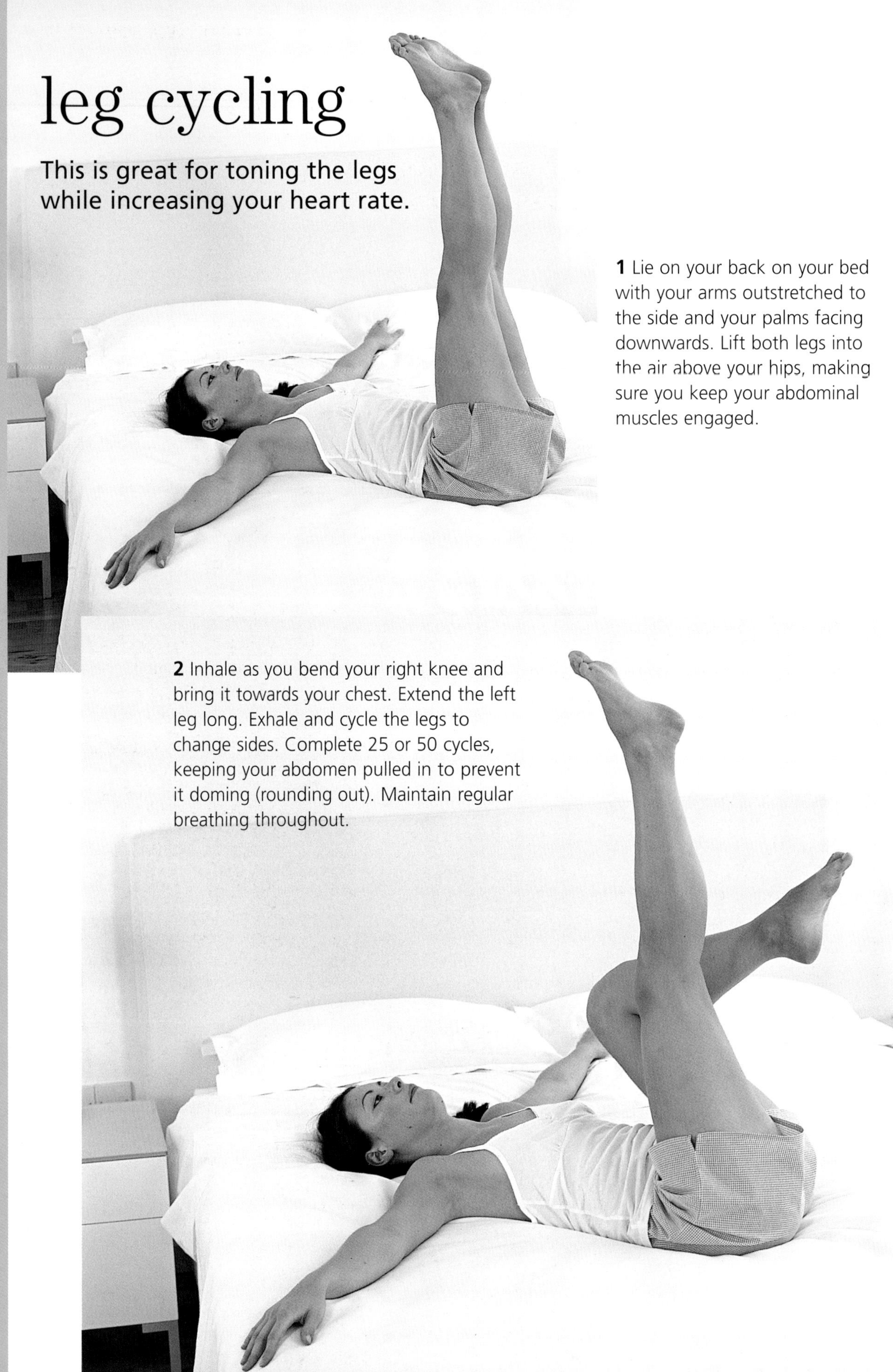

leg cycling

This is great for toning the legs while increasing your heart rate.

1 Lie on your back on your bed with your arms outstretched to the side and your palms facing downwards. Lift both legs into the air above your hips, making sure you keep your abdominal muscles engaged.

2 Inhale as you bend your right knee and bring it towards your chest. Extend the left leg long. Exhale and cycle the legs to change sides. Complete 25 or 50 cycles, keeping your abdomen pulled in to prevent it doming (rounding out). Maintain regular breathing throughout.

pulse raiser on the spot

This warms up the legs, mobilizes the ankle joints and increases the heart rate. It is deceptively hard to do.

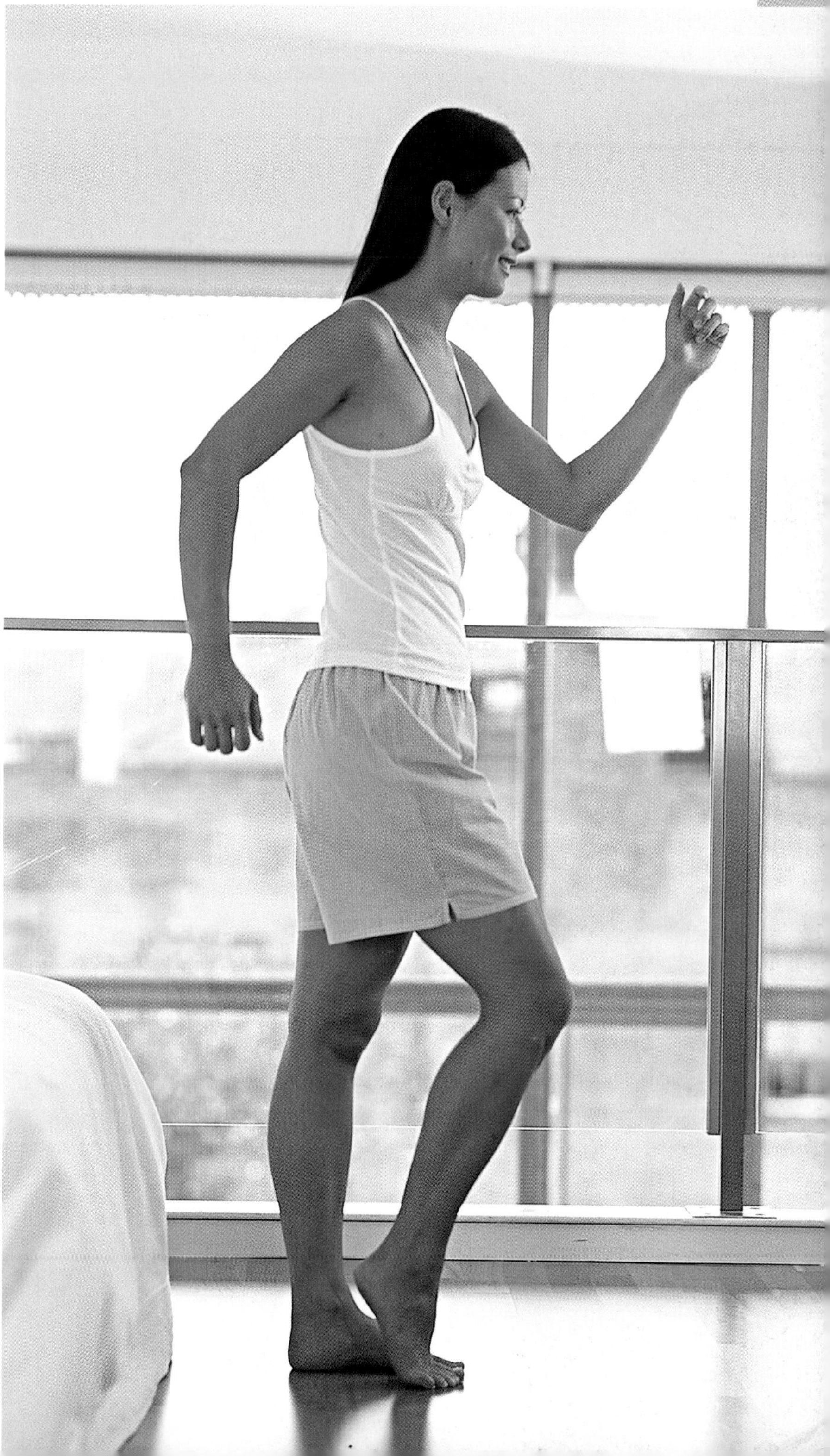

1 Stand with your feet hip width apart and your knees slightly soft. Breathing normally throughout, come up on to the balls of your feet, making sure that your body doesn't lean forwards. Now drop your left heel back down, bending your right knee over your foot as you do so. Swap legs so that you are walking on the spot. The idea is to keep lengthening upwards, all the time keeping your weight centred, your pelvis level and your waist long (thanks to full lungs and hollowed abdominals). Keep going for 3 minutes.

oxygen-pumping knee raises

This movement works across the body, toning the thighs, waist and buttock muscles while conditioning the heart and lungs.

1 Stand in a split stance with your left leg behind you, your feet hip width apart, and your arms outstretched above your head. Ensure your spine is elongated, your chest open and your weight evenly distributed across both feet. Inhale while lifting your left knee and pointing it towards your right hip and at the same time pulling both arms down towards the left knee from a diagonal direction.

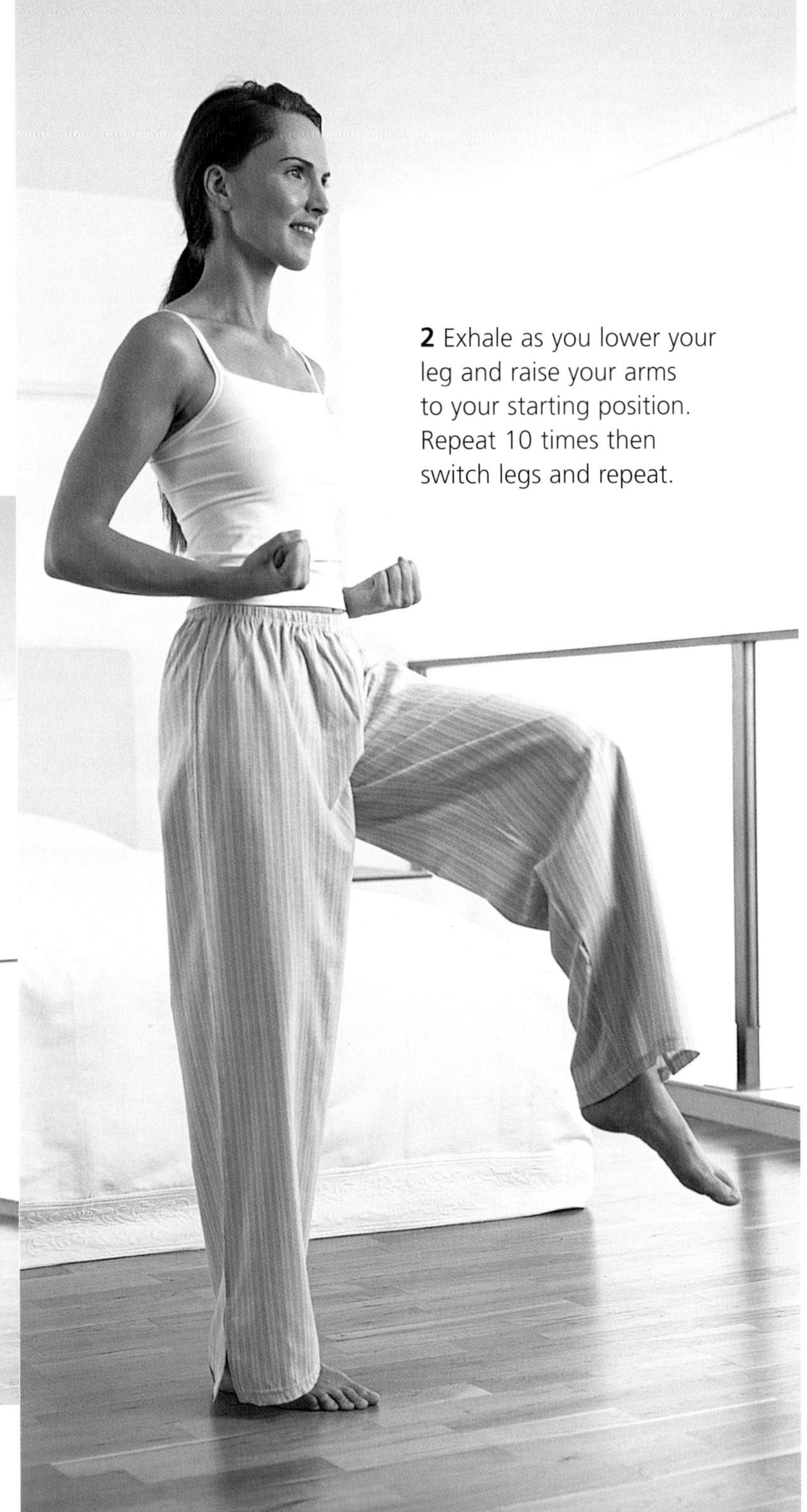

2 Exhale as you lower your leg and raise your arms to your starting position. Repeat 10 times then switch legs and repeat.

leg lunges

This heart-pumping exercise is great for strengthening your legs, spine and abdominals. It will also tone your buttocks and thighs.

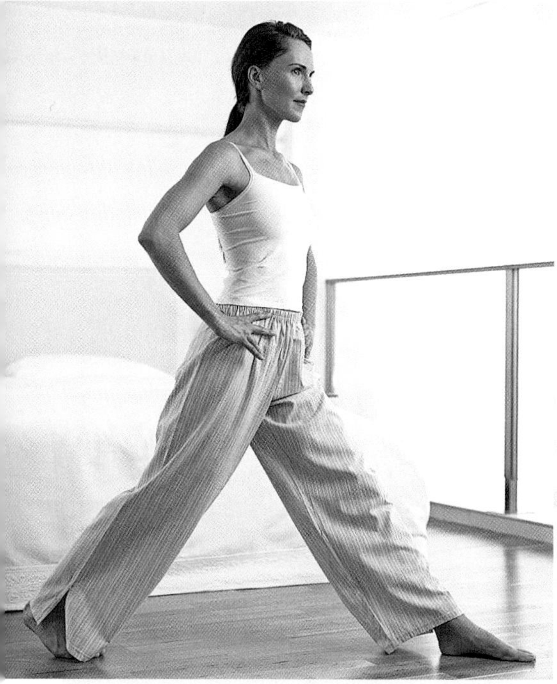

1 Stand tall with one leg forward, the foot flat on the floor, and the other leg behind you with the heel off the floor. Use a window ledge or banisters for support if necessary. Ensure your spine is long and your abdominal muscles engaged; your shoulders should be down and your neck long, away from your shoulders.

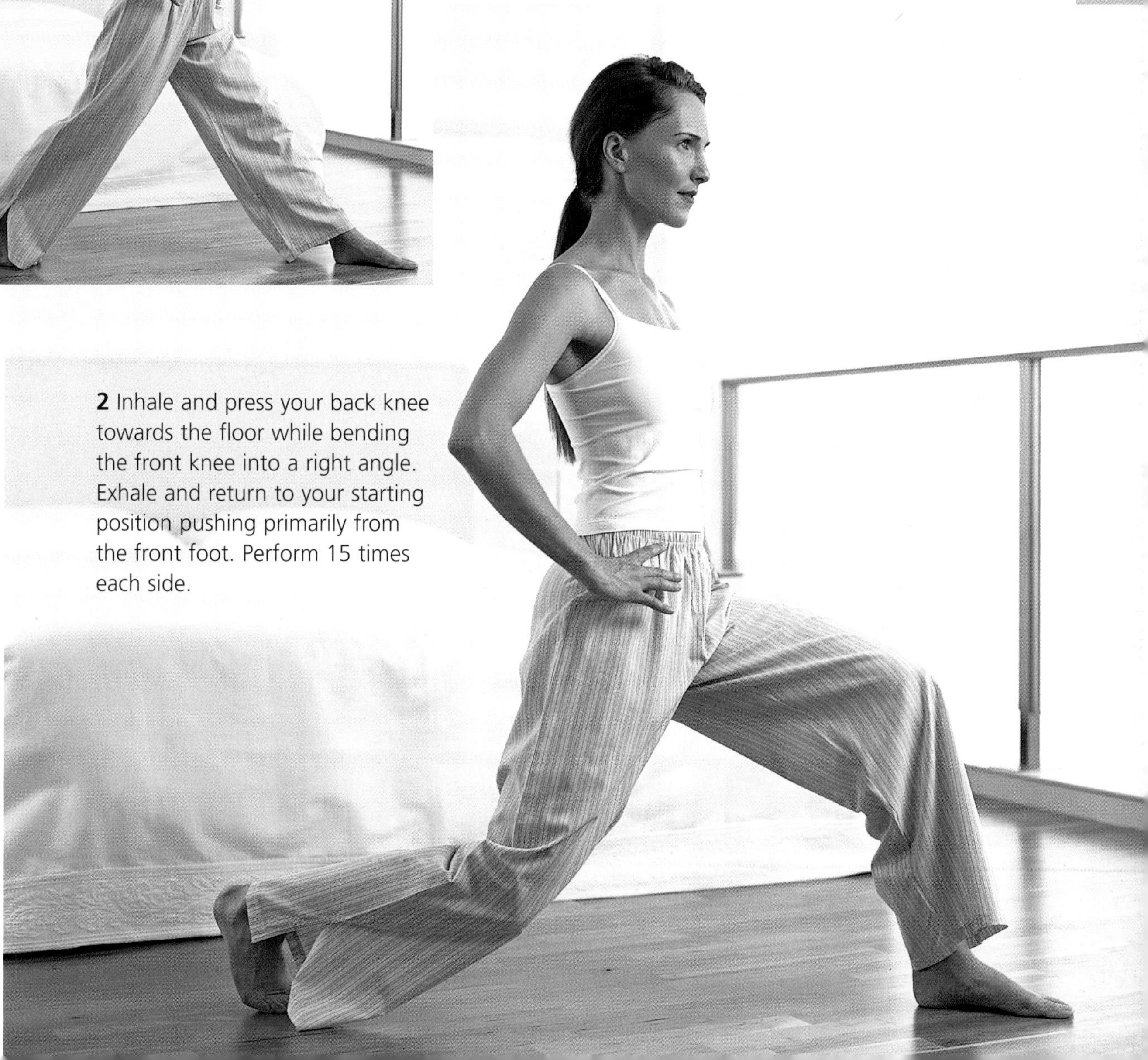

2 Inhale and press your back knee towards the floor while bending the front knee into a right angle. Exhale and return to your starting position pushing primarily from the front foot. Perform 15 times each side.

butt toners

Use steps to tone your calves, legs and buttocks, while at the same time conditioning your spine.

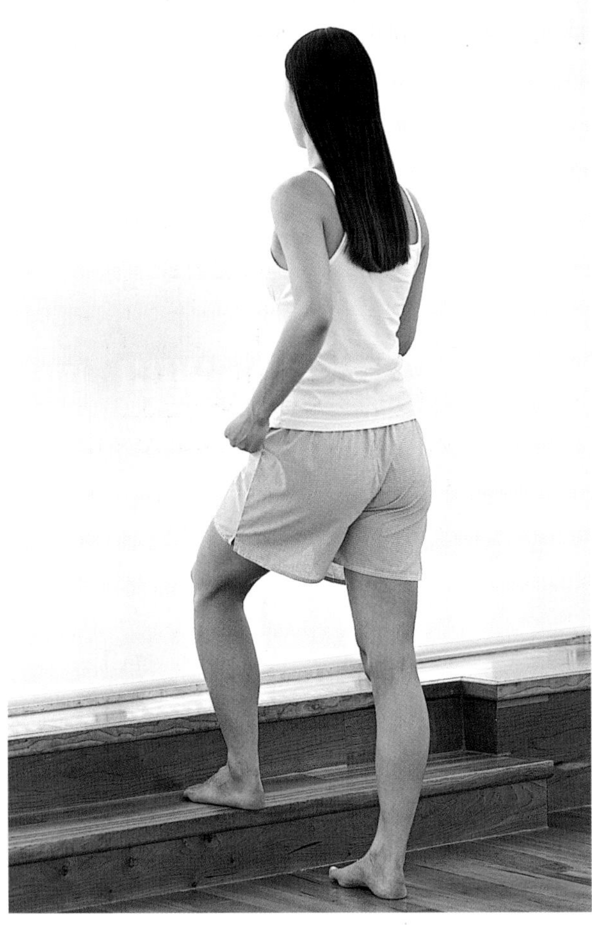

1 Stand in front of a staircase or series of steps. Inhale while stepping up with your left foot on to the first or second step. Keep your spine long and your abdomen hollow. Take care to land with your foot perfectly balanced – try not to roll from ball to foot, as you will overwork your calf muscles.

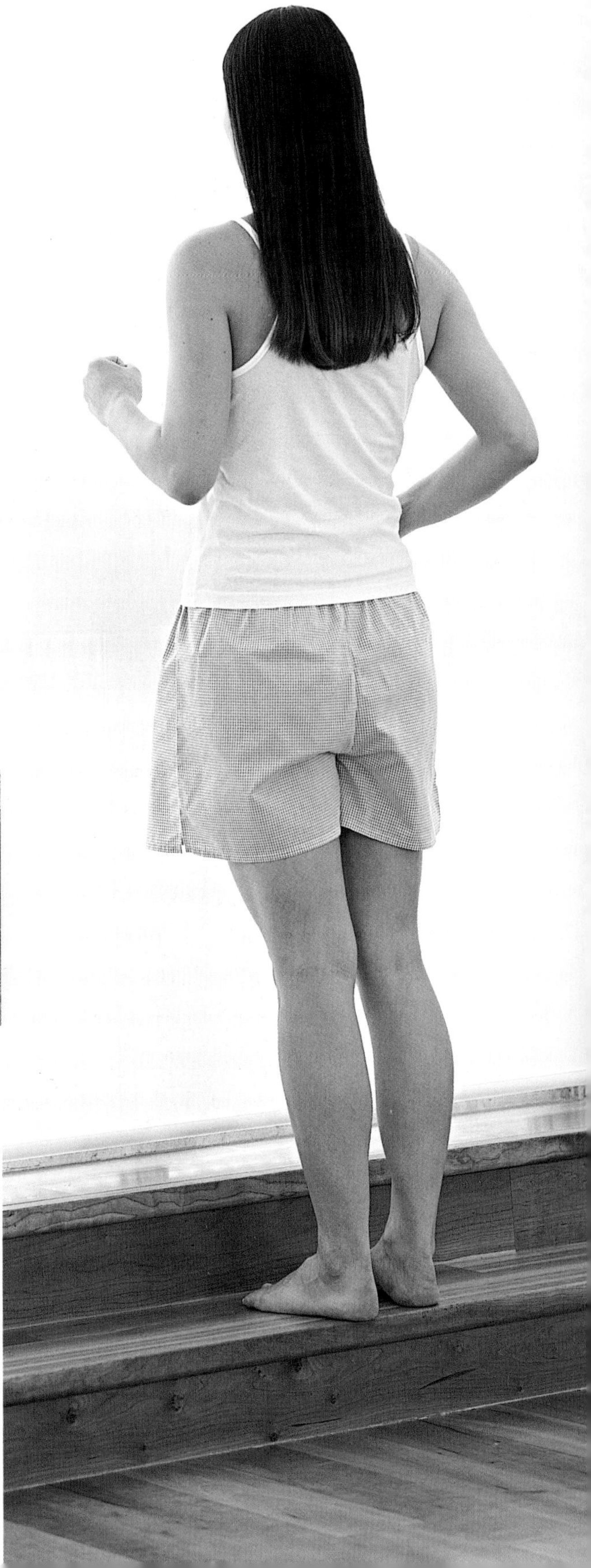

2 Exhale and step up with the other foot. Stand erect with your chest broad.

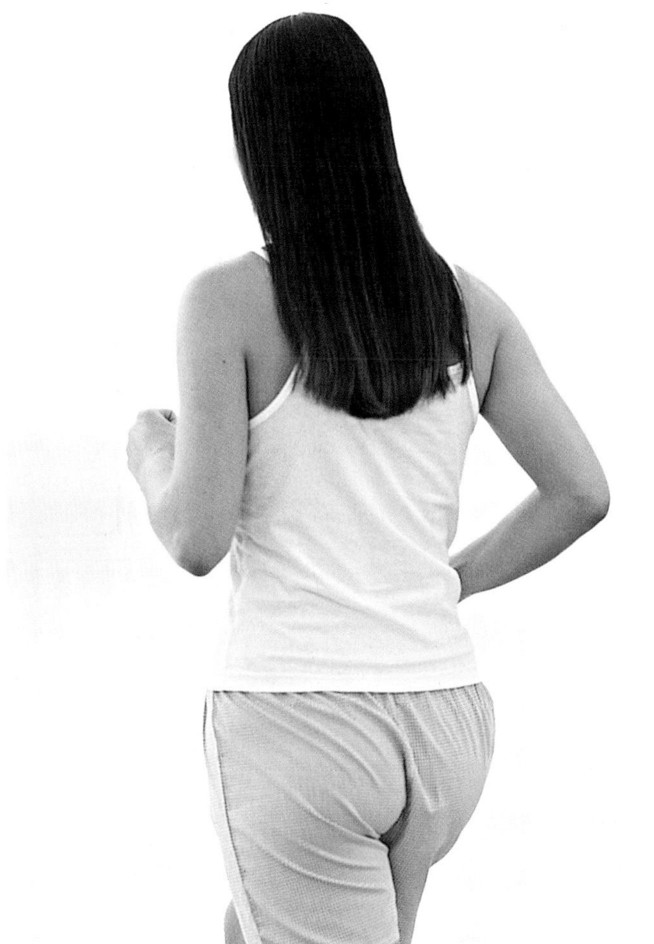

3 Inhale and lightly step down with your left foot.

4 Exhale and return to your starting position in front of the staircase. Repeat the sequence a total of 25–50 times, perhaps increasing the number of steps you use at a time to make your legs stretch further.

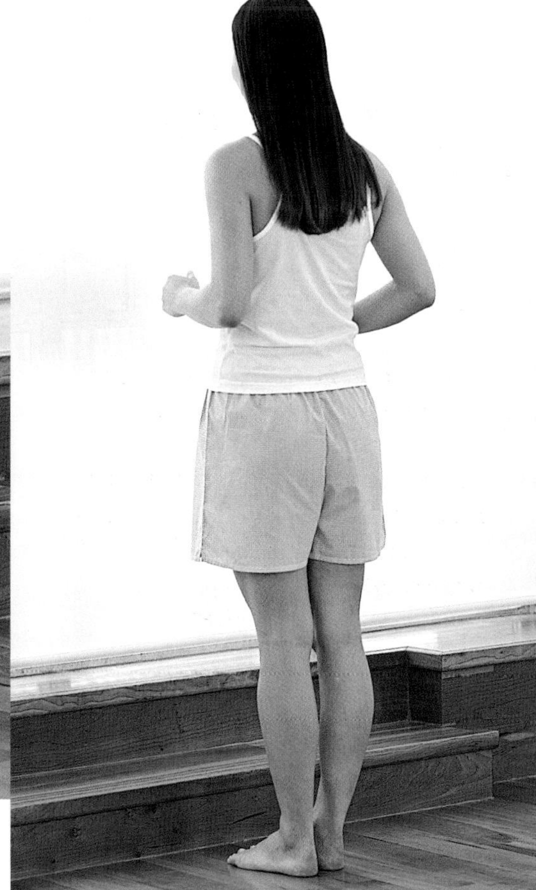

body sculpting

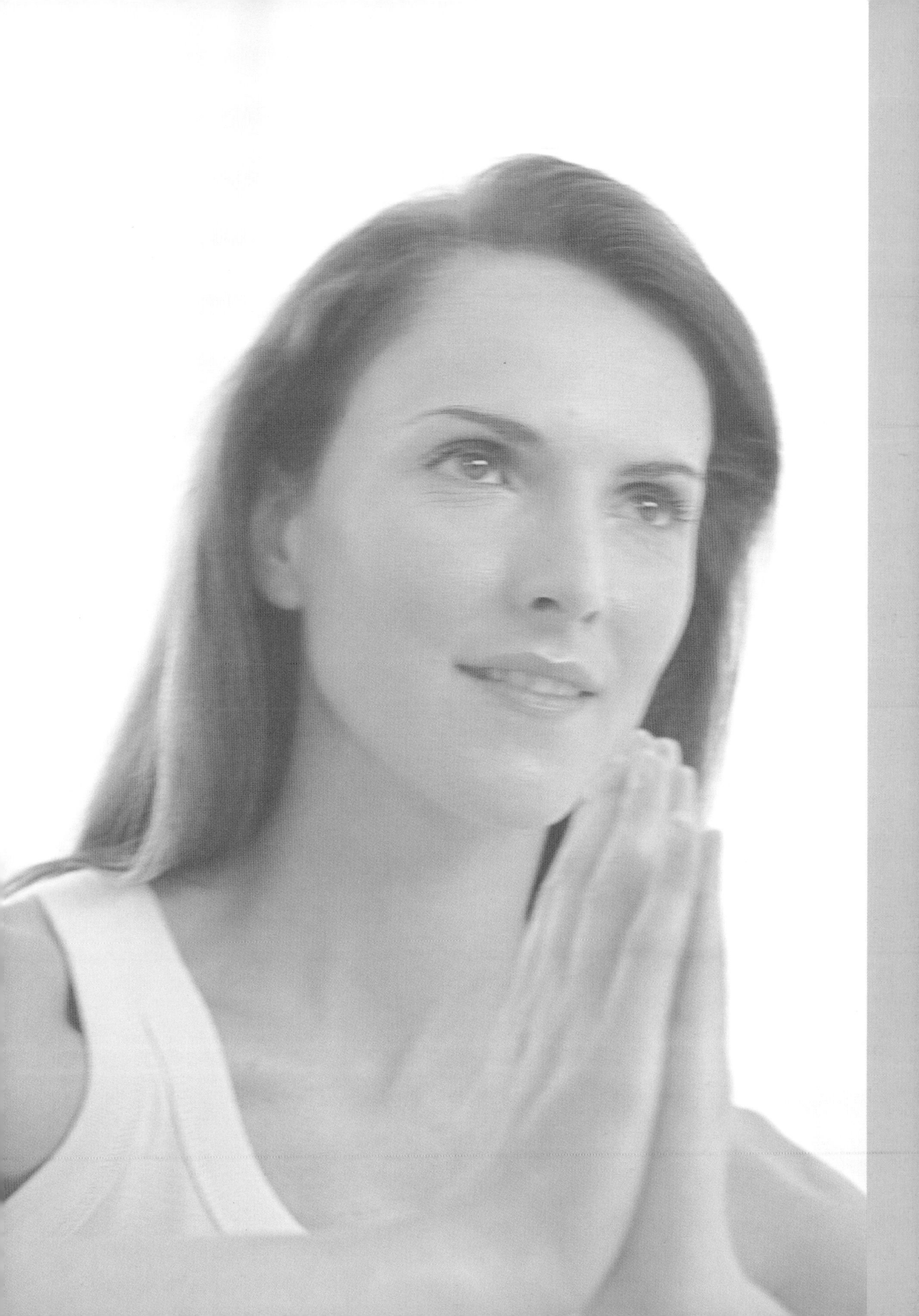

body sculpting

The body sculpting workout focuses on strengthening specific muscle groups to improve their tone and condition. This is achieved by contracting the belly of the muscles during movement to strengthen, and ultimately tone, muscles by building up muscle fibres. Exercises that use your bodyweight to provide resistance, such as the 'Triceps dips' and 'Ledge press-ups', work the muscles even harder and are therefore even more effective.

Benefits

The benefits of body sculpting are manifold. Toned muscles not only make us look more shapely and feel better, they also increase our metabolism, which is especially important for keeping weight under control as we get older. Muscle is very active tissue and the natural loss of muscle as we age leads to a lower energy requirement and therefore a reduced resting metabolism. In other words we burn less calories while resting.

Another very good reason for body sculpting is that good muscle tone goes hand in hand with stronger bones. Research has shown that regular weight-bearing exercise stimulates bone strengthening and helps prevent osteoporosis, so the sooner you start body sculpting the better.

'Bone-loading exercises are the best ones to beat osteoporosis'

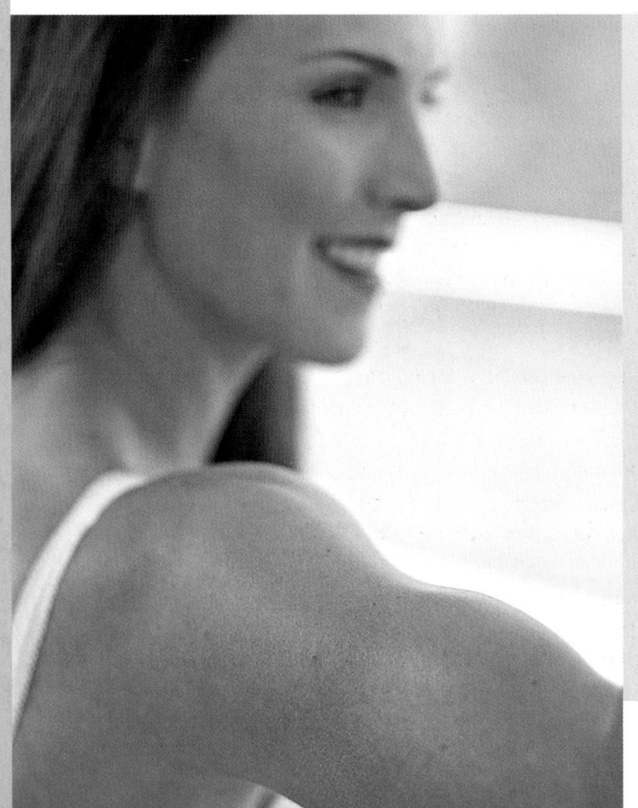

BENEFITS OF BODY SCULPTING

- Increased muscle and bone strength
- Higher metabolism
- Improved posture and appearance
- Reduced body fat
- More overall energy

'Regular body sculpting can improve muscle tissue and enhance the way you look and feel'

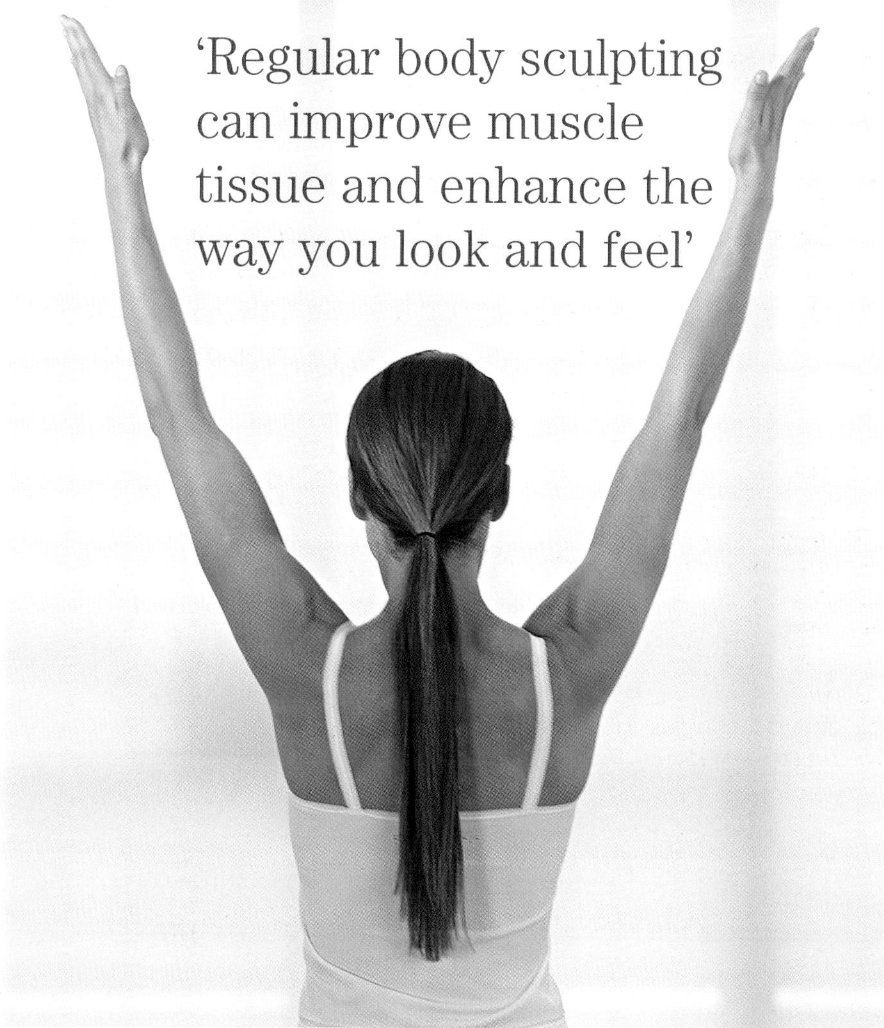

Osteoporosis

Osteoporosis is a weakening of the bones, which can lead to breaks that are difficult to heal – hence its alternative name, brittle bone disease. It is sometimes referred to as the silent disease as often people do not know they have it until it is diagnosed following a fracture. Everyone is potentially at risk of suffering osteoporosis because it is a natural part of the ageing process that bones become weaker and their inner 'honeycomb' of collagen, blood vessels and bone marrow less dense. However, plenty of exercise and a well-balanced, calcium-rich diet, especially in childhood and adolescence when the bones are growing, help prevent the disease.

According to the UK's National Osteoporosis Society, osteoporosis affects one in three women and one in 12 men over the age of 50. Women are particularly at risk because they have smaller, more fragile bones to start with. This is complicated by the menopause, during which the body stops producing oestrogen – a hormone essential for good bone health. There is also research to suggest that younger women, particularly those who are underweight or who have suffered anorexia, are likely candidates for the disease.

The 10-minute body sculpting wake-up workout includes bone-loading exercises to offset osteoporosis, but it must be made clear that once you have the disease exercise does not necessarily get rid of it. If you are in any doubt about your own body you must consult a physician before embarking on an exercise programme.

morning prayer squats

This squat will strengthen legs, ankles and feet, but do not try it if you suffer from back pain or knee problems.

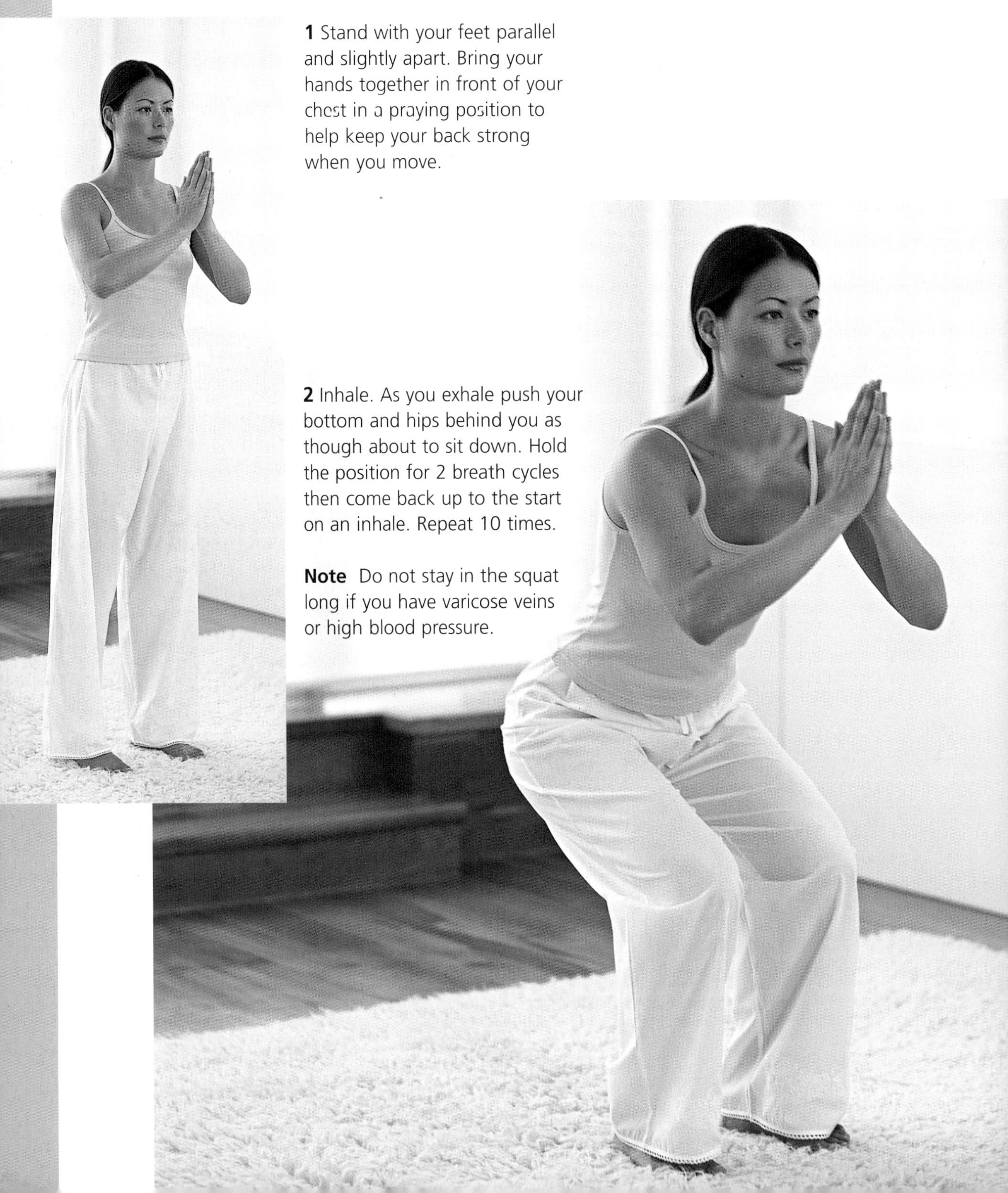

1 Stand with your feet parallel and slightly apart. Bring your hands together in front of your chest in a praying position to help keep your back strong when you move.

2 Inhale. As you exhale push your bottom and hips behind you as though about to sit down. Hold the position for 2 breath cycles then come back up to the start on an inhale. Repeat 10 times.

Note Do not stay in the squat long if you have varicose veins or high blood pressure.

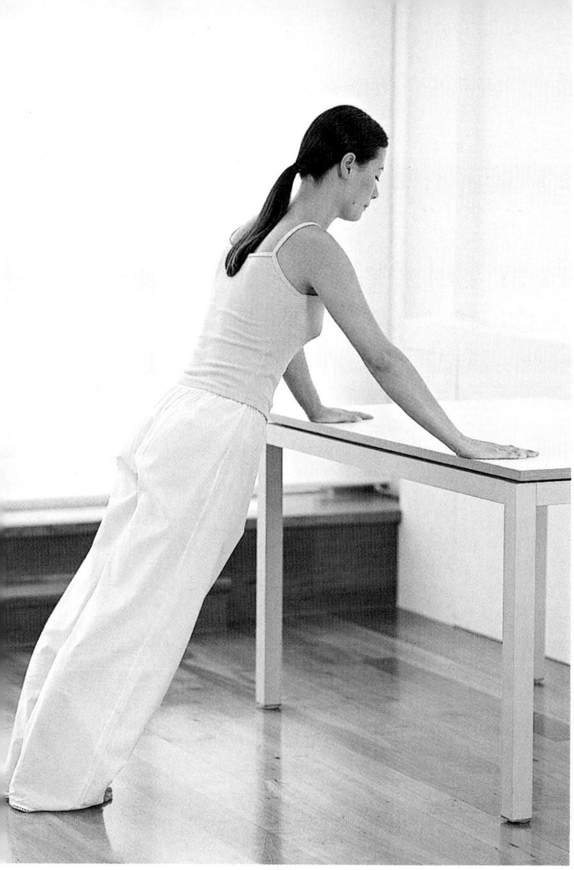

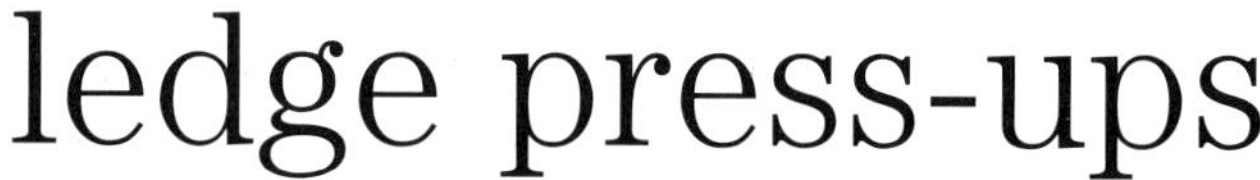

ledge press-ups

Strengthen your shoulders, chest and upper arms with these standing press-ups.

1 Stand a comfortable distance from a window ledge or sturdy table. Place your hands on the support, one-and-a-half times your shoulders width apart. Walk your feet further away from the support.

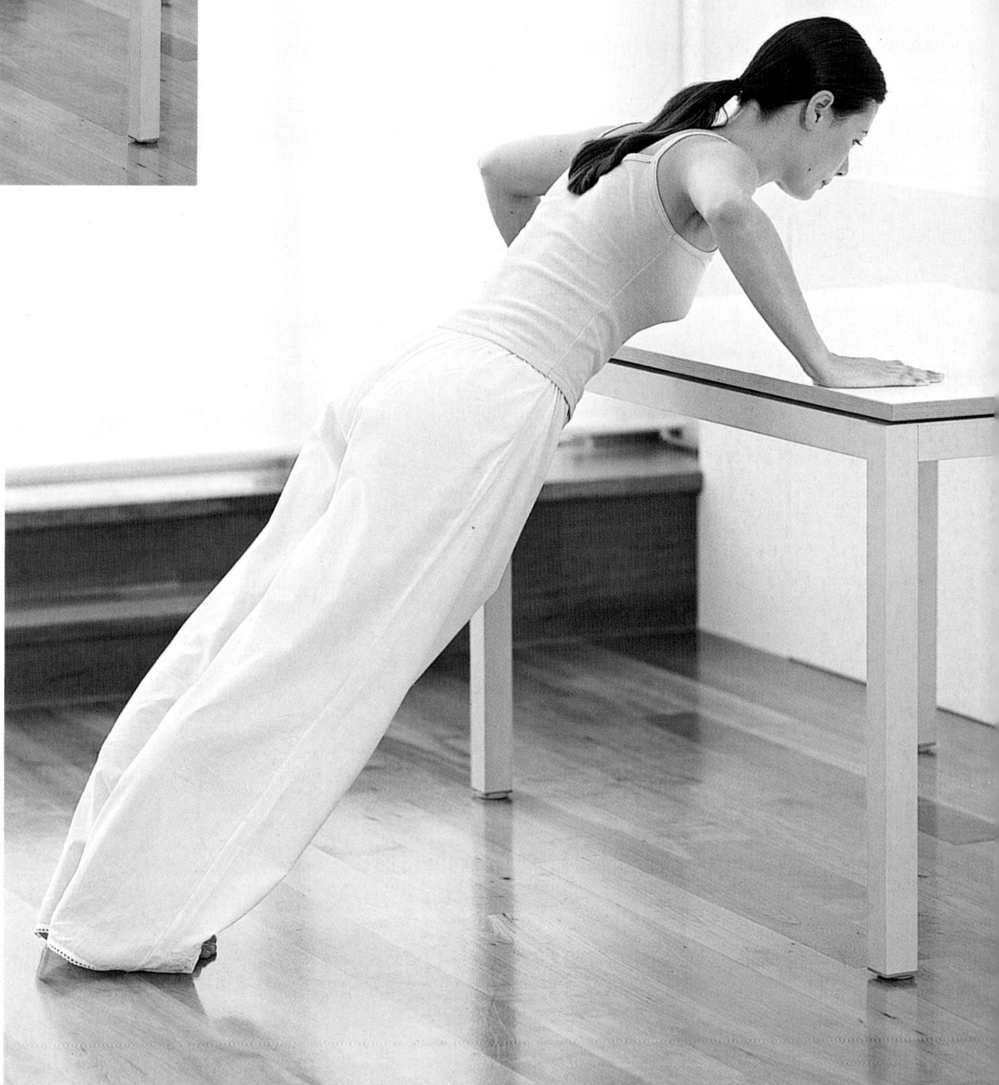

2 Inhale. As you exhale bend your elbows and press your trunk towards the window ledge – the further your legs are from the support, the harder the exercise will be. Inhale as you push your trunk away from the ledge back to your starting position. Repeat 10 times, following the correct breathing pattern.

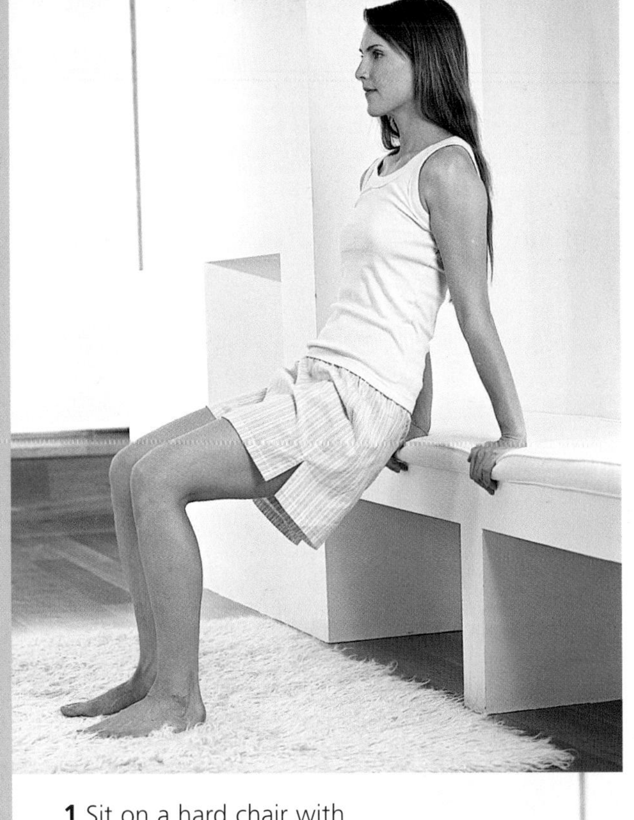

triceps dips

Dips tone the triceps muscles, firming up any soft tissue around the back of the upper arms.

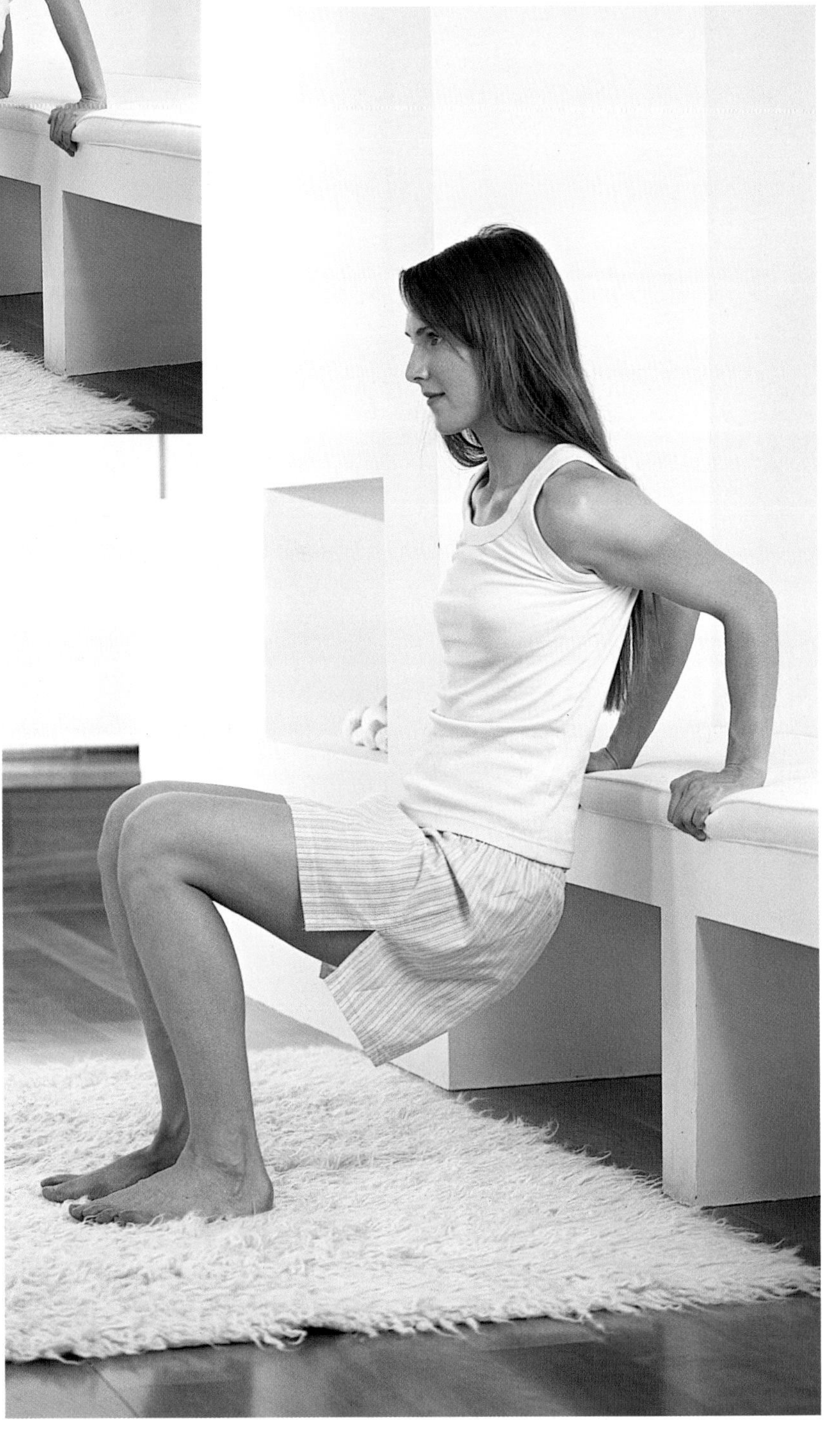

1 Sit on a hard chair with your hands palms down and gripping the chair seat, and your feet flat on the floor. Ensure your spine is erect and your abdomen engaged. Slide your bottom forwards off the edge of the seat so that you are supporting yourself with your arms but do not lock your elbows.

2 Inhale. As you exhale, bend your elbows, ensuring they point behind you rather than to the side, and lower your body until your arms are at right angles. Inhale and push back to your starting position. Repeat 15 times, following the correct breathing pattern.

buttocks bridging

This exercise tones the buttocks and thighs and releases the spine. It increases circulation and nourishes the nervous system.

1 Lie on your back on the floor and place your lower legs on the edge of a low bed or chair. Place your arms down by your sides.

2 Inhale. As you exhale push your pelvis upwards to lift your lower spine and middle back off the floor. Rest gently on your upper shoulders, but avoid applying pressure to your neck. Inhale and drop your pelvis slightly. As you exhale lift your pelvis and squeeze your buttocks together. Repeat 20 times, following the correct breathing pattern.

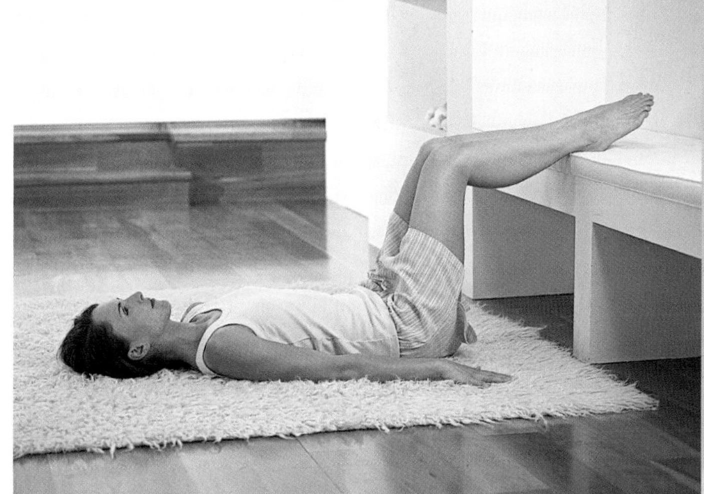

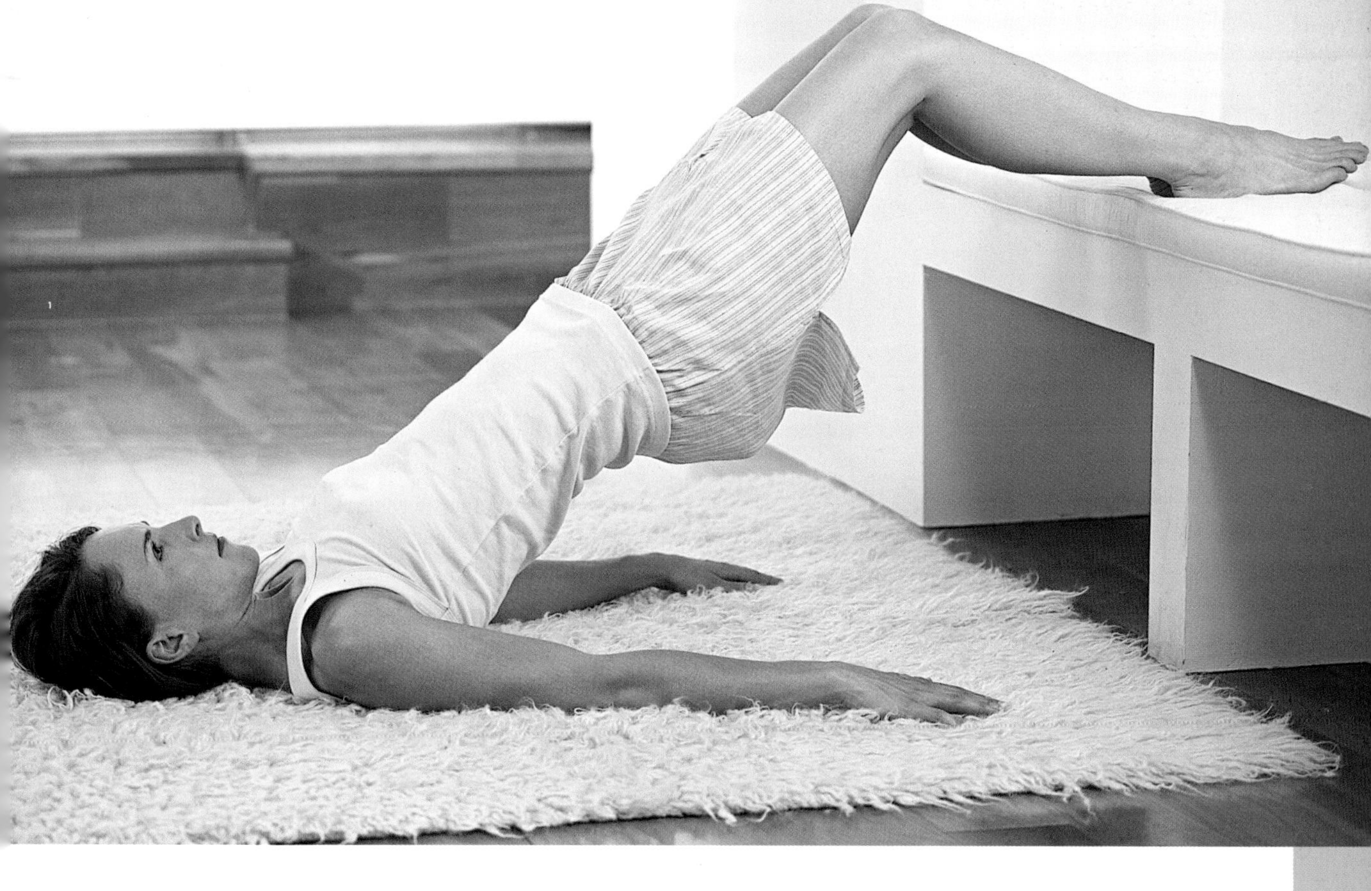

spine raises

This movement helps to maintain a healthy spine and strong abdomen.

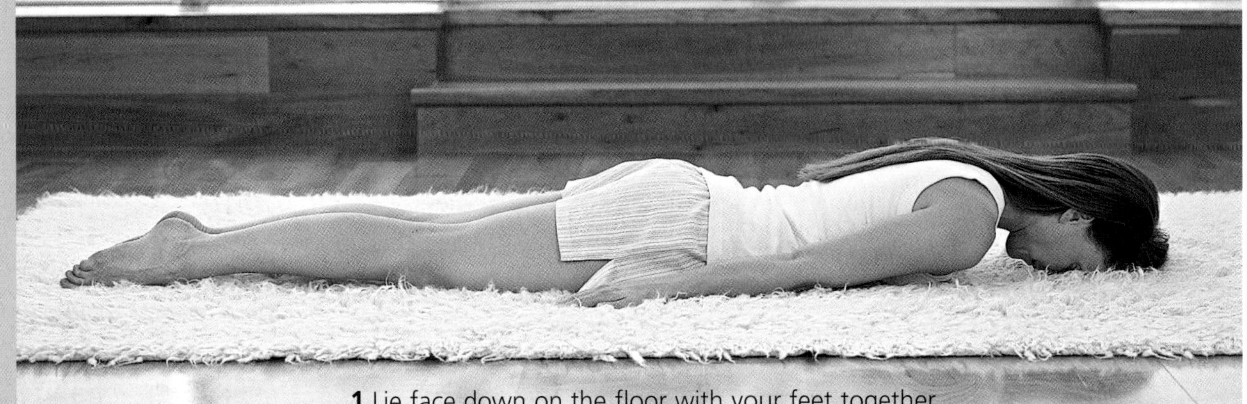

1 Lie face down on the floor with your feet together, your arms down by your sides and your palms facing downwards. Ensure your neck is in line with your spine and draw in your thigh and abdominal muscles.

2 Inhale. As you exhale lift your trunk and legs away from the floor. Ensure your abdomen stays hollow – if you feel it doming (rounding out), do not lift your trunk and legs so high. Inhale gently as you release back towards the floor, but do not rest on it completely. Repeat 10 times, breathing slowly.

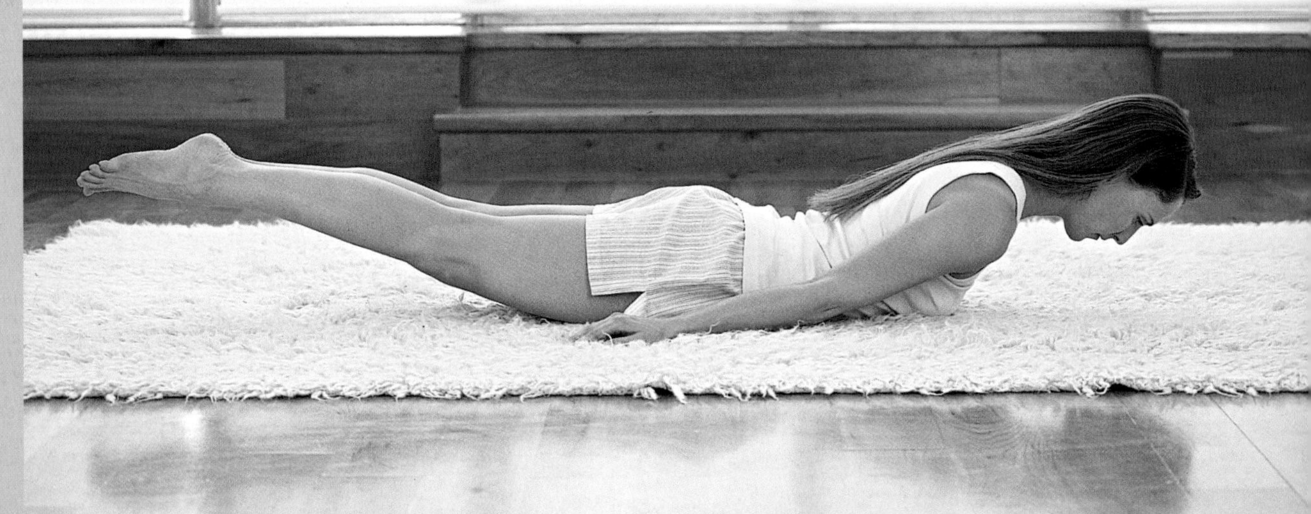

hamstring curls

Hold a rolled-up towel between your lower legs to tone the muscles that run up the back of your thighs.

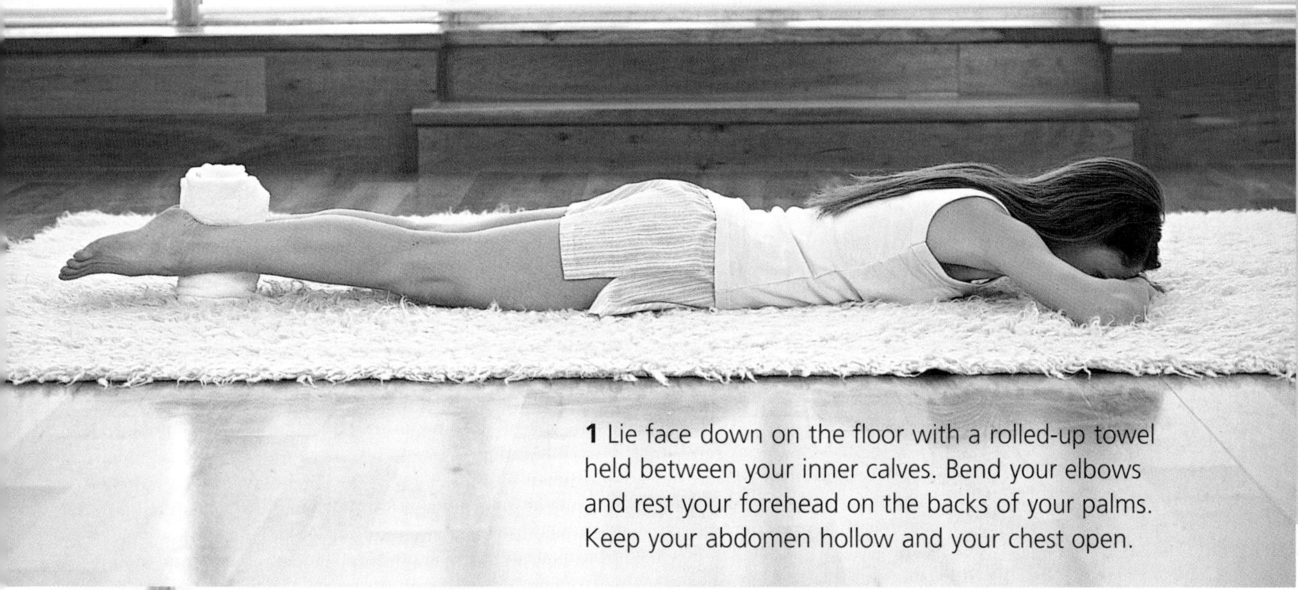

1 Lie face down on the floor with a rolled-up towel held between your inner calves. Bend your elbows and rest your forehead on the backs of your palms. Keep your abdomen hollow and your chest open.

2 Inhale. As you exhale bend your knees and draw your ankles towards your buttocks, keeping your hips pressed into the floor as you do so. Inhale as you straighten your legs again but don't let them completely relax. Pull your thigh muscles into the thigh bones to tone the legs. Repeat 12 times with the correct breathing pattern.

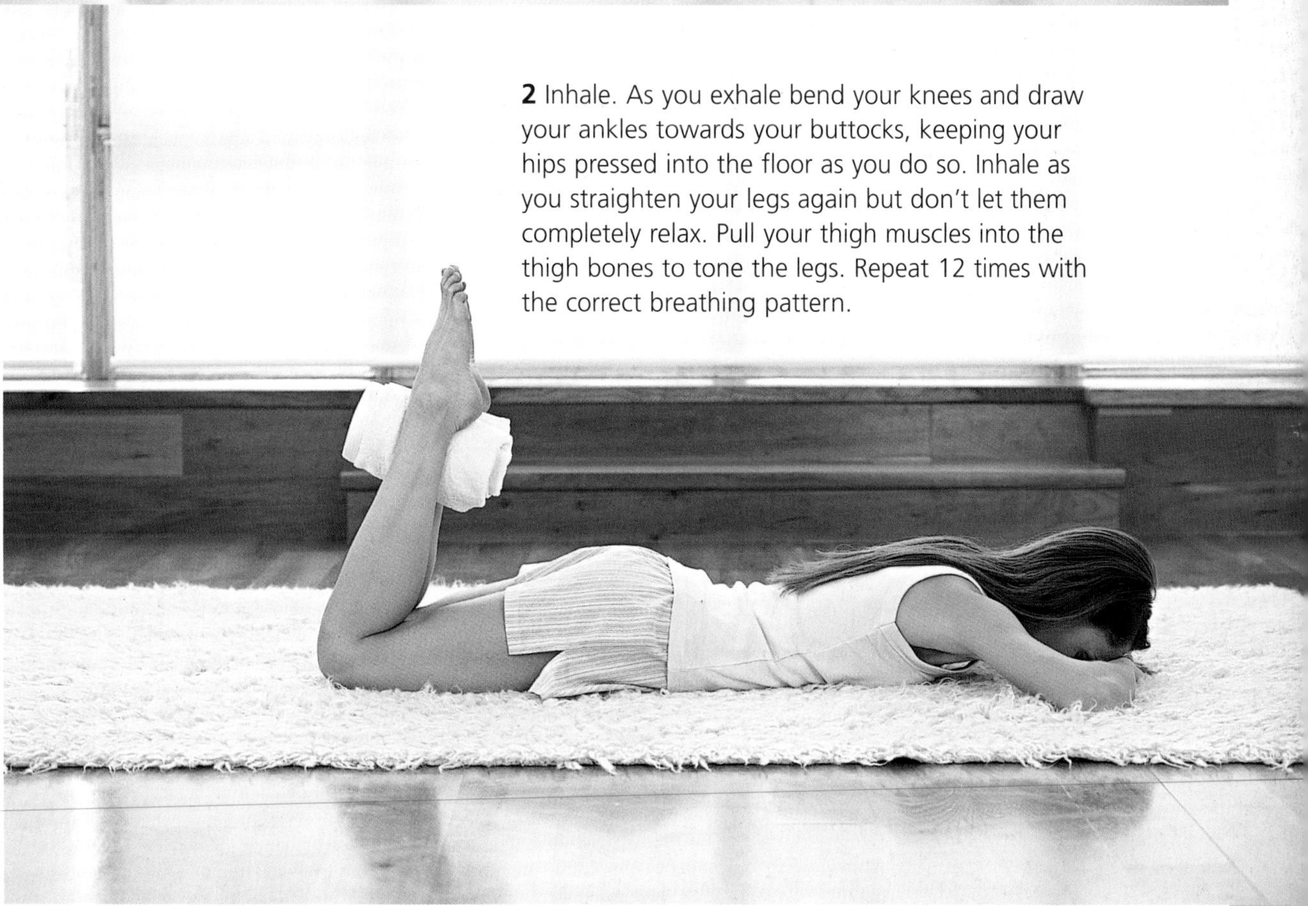

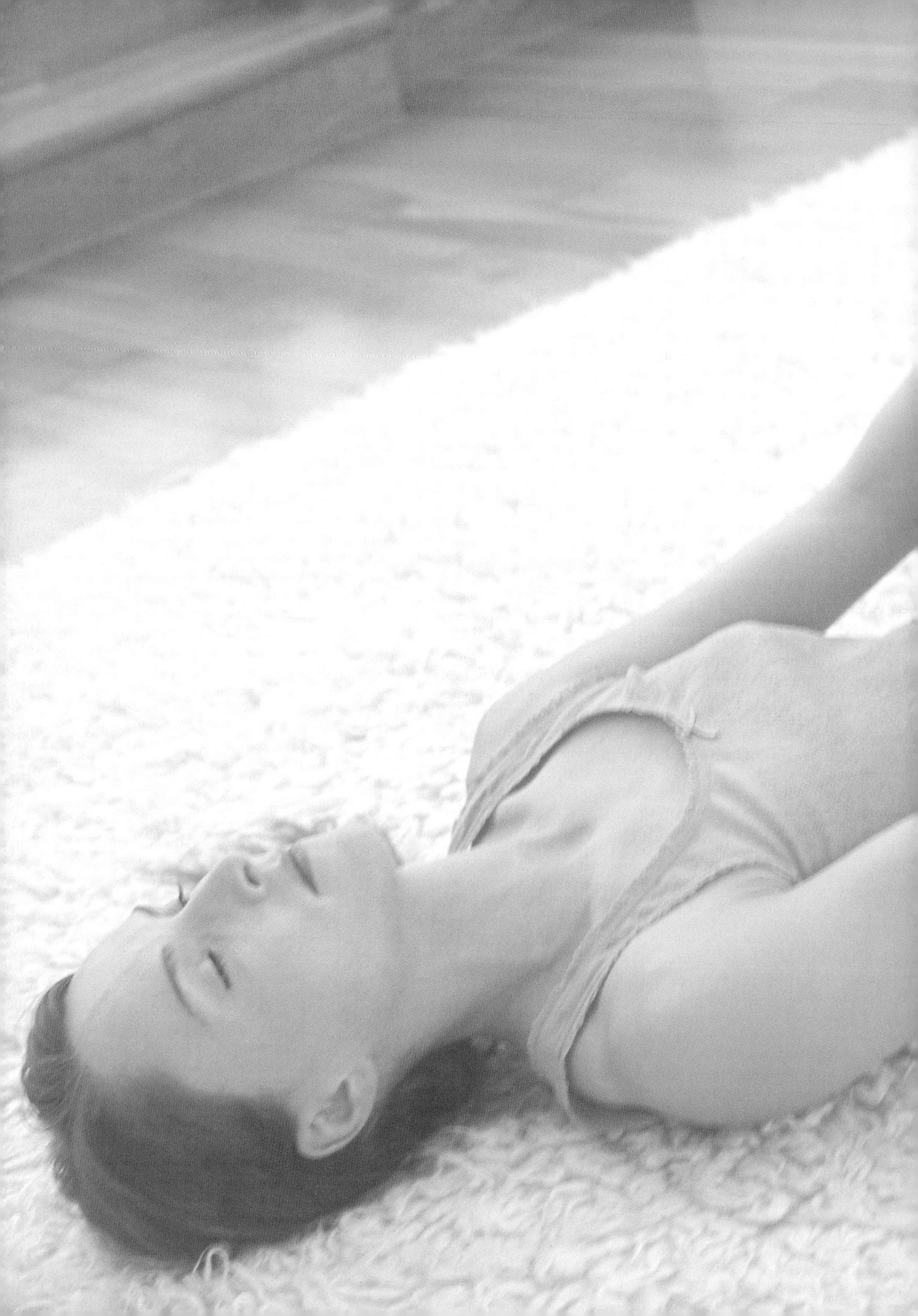

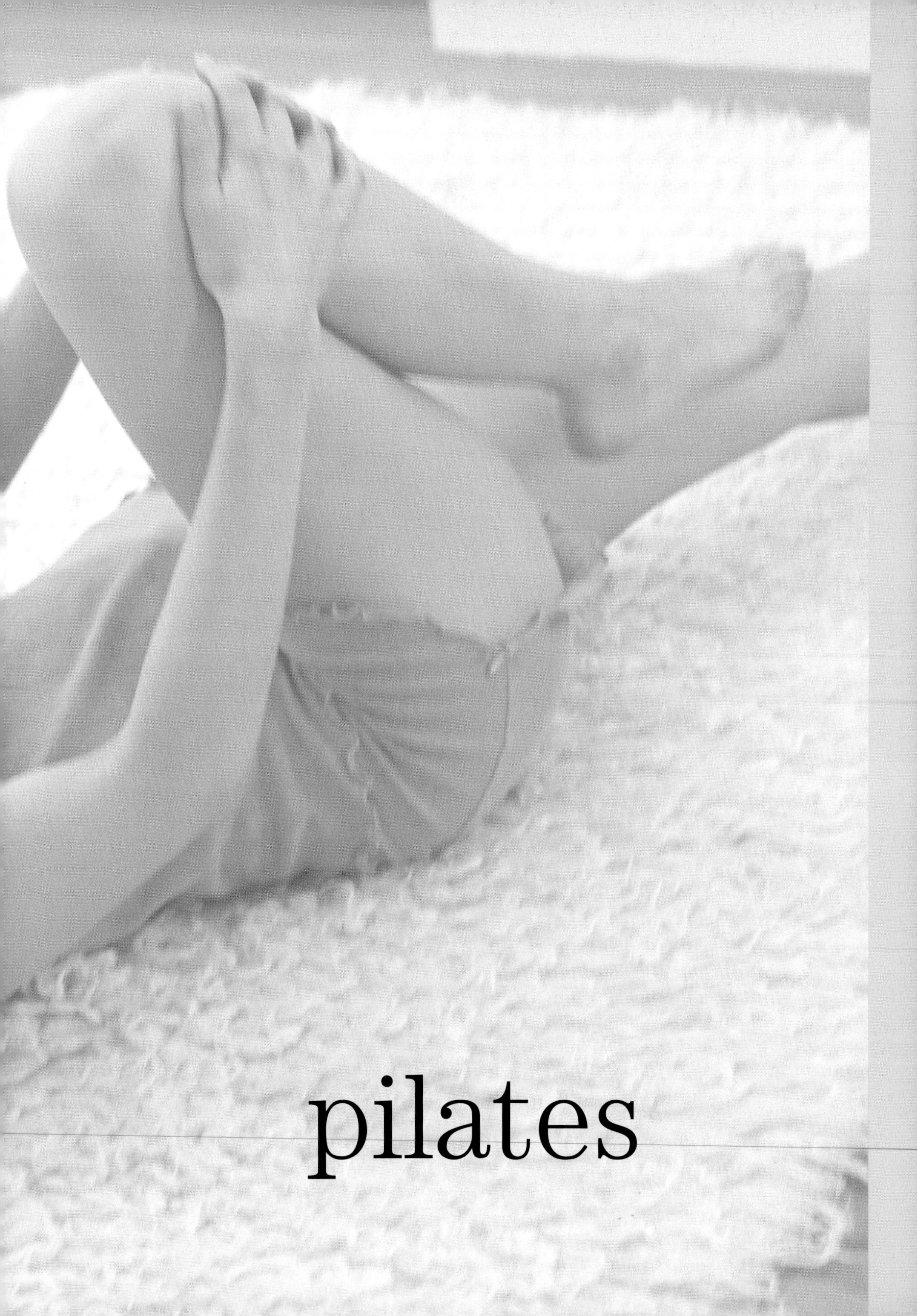

pilates

pilates

Most exercise programmes lack one basic ingredient: balance. Weight training, for example, maximizes muscular strength, and cardiovascular exercise increases stamina. Pilates exercises, however, focus on balancing the actions of the body's whole structure – the skeleton, joints, muscles and major organs – and strengthening the core (the body's trunk).

What is it?

The Pilates system was developed by Joseph Hubertus Pilates in the early 20th century to overcome his own poor physical health. Its principles focus on improving health, overall strength, postural realignment and the immune system. Pilates denounced the flat feet and curved spines he saw around him, the postural defects caused by poorly designed furniture, and the unbalanced exercises of other physical trainers, which distorted the body. The association between physical and mental wellbeing was his guiding principle and modern-day Pilates still aims for the coordination of body and mind through exercise.

Pilates is suitable for all levels of fitness and is a good basis for all the exercise sections in this wake-up workout programme. Many people have adopted it as a way to include exercise in their everyday lives. Pilates can have a positive impact in a number of ways (see box below) and is particularly suitable for those with weaknesses around the spine or hips who find regular activities difficult.

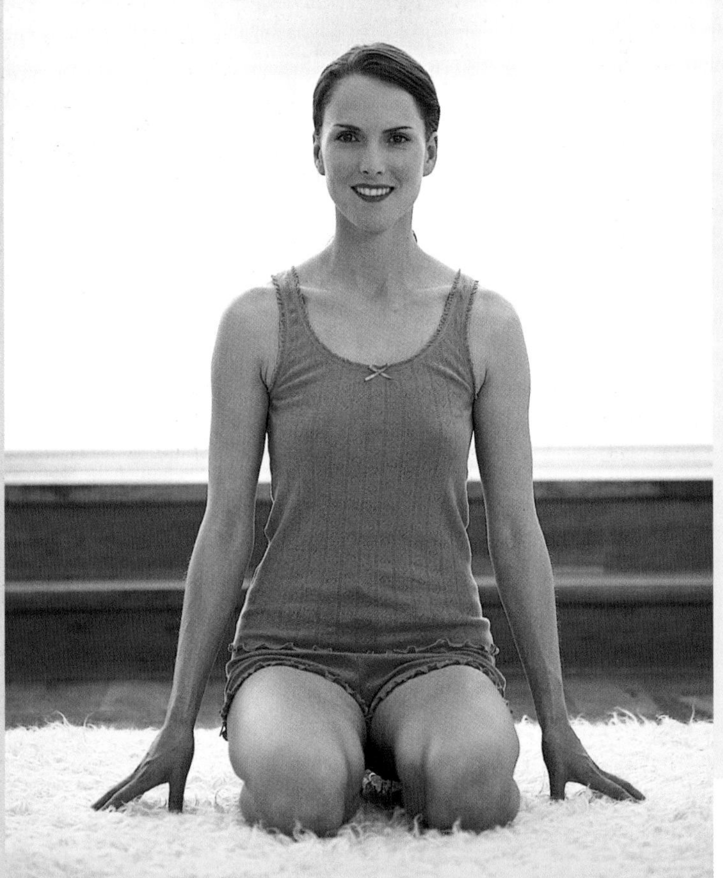

BENEFITS OF PILATES

- Increased muscle tone without bulk
- Longer and leaner look
- Increased energy
- Improved balance
- Reduced stress
- Better circulation
- Enhanced immune system

> 'Pilates works your abdominal and back muscles, diaphragm and pelvic floor as a unit, to create strength and stability and enhance all areas of activity'

Pelvic floor elevators

Your pelvic floor muscles run from your pubic bone through the groin to your tail bone in the lower spine. This thin sheath of muscle centres and stabilizes the abdominal organs. If it is allowed to go saggy or lose tone then the abdominal organs get pushed forwards towards the abdomen and the abdomen wall protrudes.

The following simple Pilates exercise teaches you how to zip up and tone your pelvic floor so that your abdominals remain flat and your spine supported. Keep your actions gentle and low for lumbar stability.

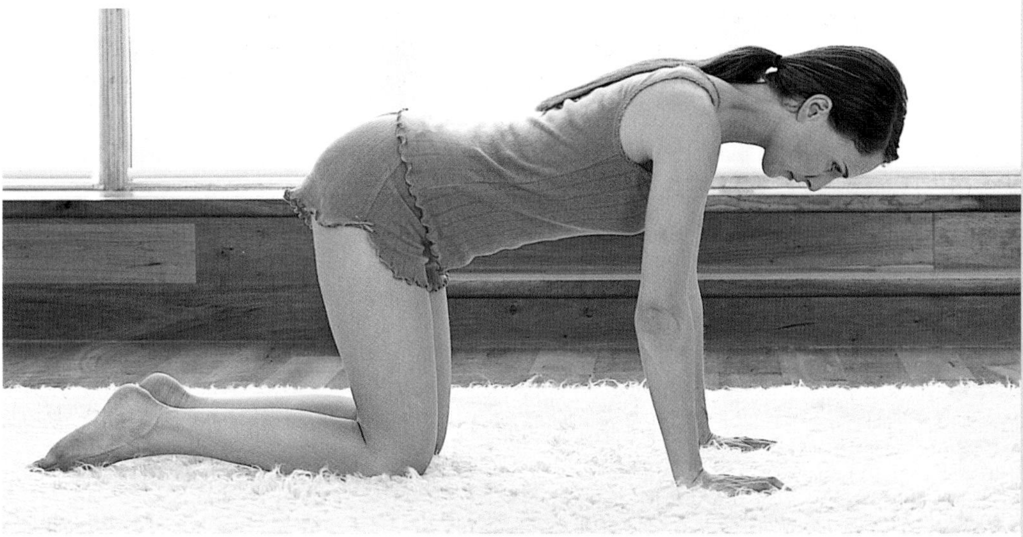

1 Kneel on all fours with your hands flat on the floor directly beneath your shoulders and your hips directly above your knees. Lengthen your head away from your sacrum (tail bone), keeping your pelvis in neutral and a natural curve in the base of your spine subtle enough to balance a tennis ball. Be careful not to arch or round your spine excessively. Inhale to prepare. Exhale and draw up your pelvic floor muscles by 10 per cent as though to stop yourself from emptying your bladder.

2 Breathe in and breathe out and draw your pelvic floor muscles up by another 10 per cent. Inhale and exhale and, if you can, repeat one more time. Hold on to this 30 per cent engagement in your pelvic floor muscles for the duration of the exercise.

3 Now repeat the breathing but try to keep your pelvic floor muscles zipped up. After five cycles of breathing, inhale and release your pelvic floor. Exhale and rest.

balance rotations

This movement uses spine rotation and balance to improve lumbar stability.

1 Stand with your feet together (or hip width apart if you have a problem with your balance). Adopt a neutral stance with your arms engaged by your sides and your pelvic floor engaged by 20–30 per cent. Keep your shoulders back and relaxed and your face soft with your neck elongated.

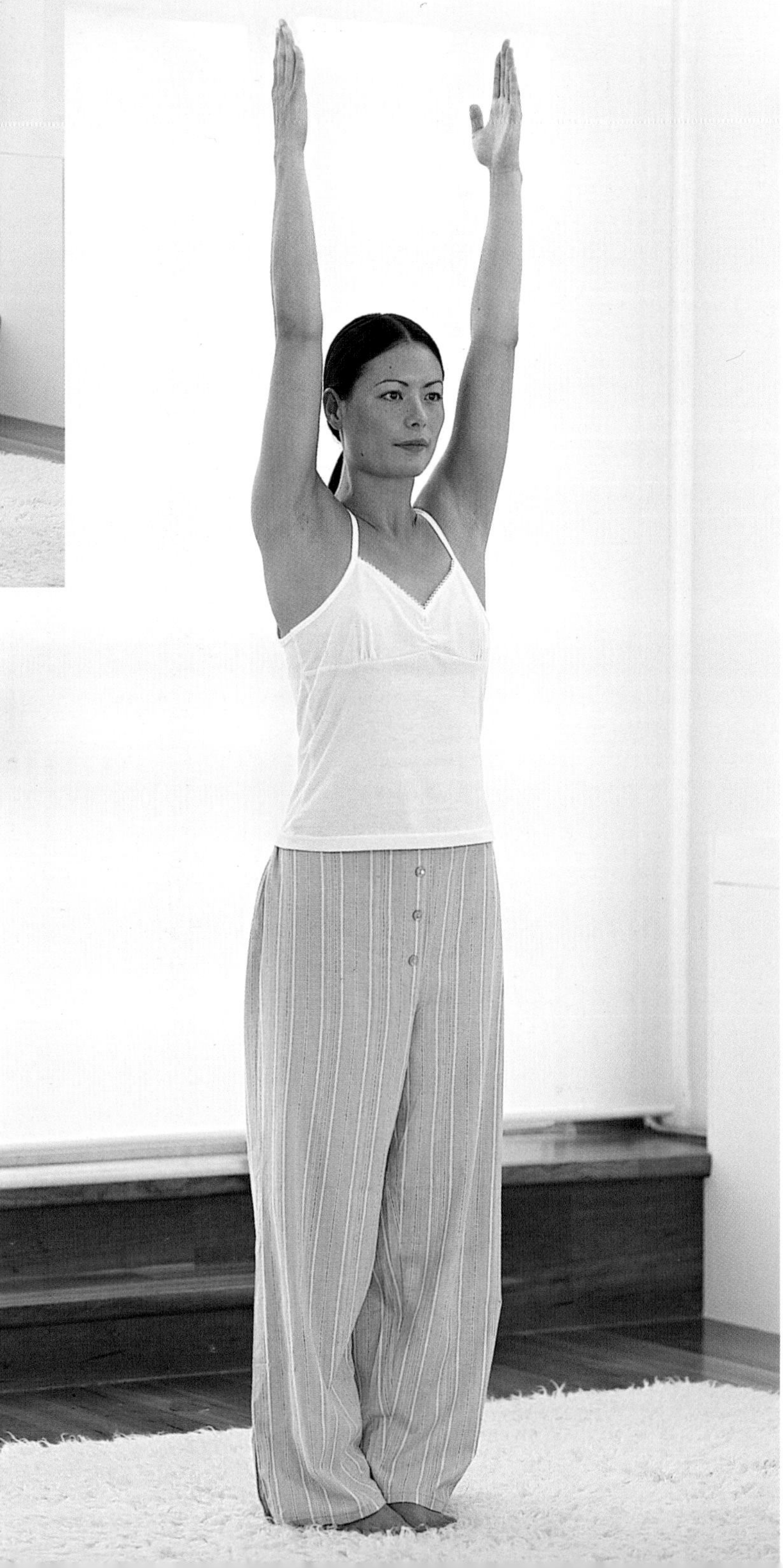

2 Breathe in and raise both arms above your head, keeping your shoulder blades down and away from your ears so as to lengthen your neck.

3 As you inhale, lift your right knee to a comfortable level and broaden your rib cage. Draw your navel in towards your spine as you lift your knee to provide maximum stability for your core. Breathe out and as you do so, bring your arms down to shoulder height with your left arm in front of you and the right arm behind you. As you extend your arms rotate your spine towards the right, feeling a small twisting sensation in your trunk. Keep your pelvic floor engaged by 20–30 per cent and keep the right knee slightly bent if it helps you to stay stable. Note, you can initially use a chair for support to help build your strength and ensure you maintain a neutral spine.

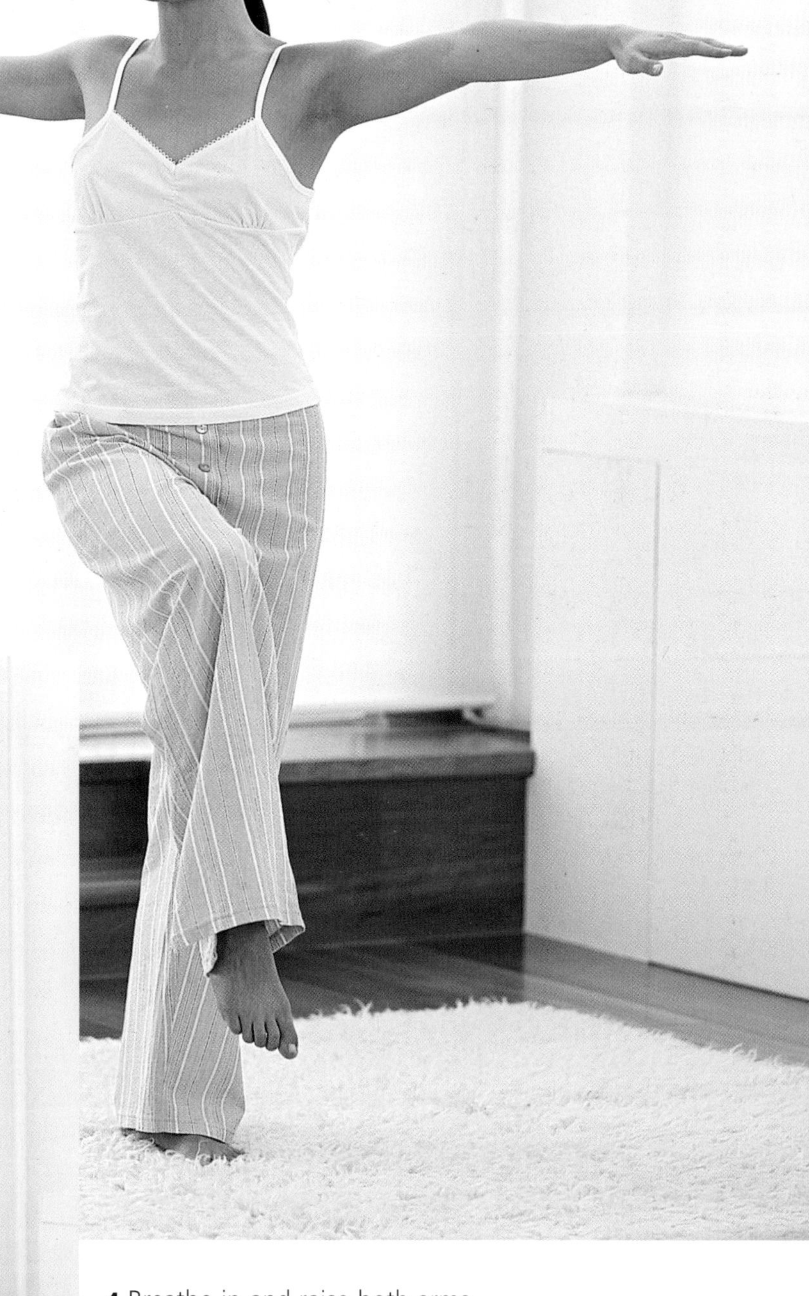

4 Breathe in and raise both arms above your head as you release your knee. Breathe out and release your arms and leg back down to the neutral starting position. Repeat 8–10 times with each leg.

lunge and balance

This strengthening movement incorporates balance while toning the thighs and reinforcing a neutral spine.

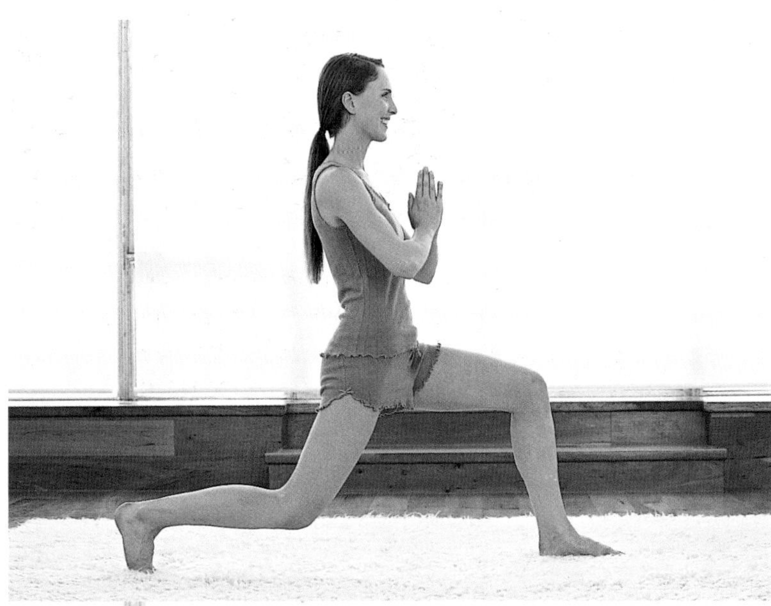

1 Stand with your left leg forwards and your right leg back, its heel off the floor. Keep your spine neutral and engage your pelvic floor by 20–30 per cent. Your ears, shoulders and hips should stay in line. Inhale and bend through both knees to bring your front knee into a right angle. Keep your pelvic floor and abdominal muscles engaged.

2 Breathe out and press your weight through your front foot to lift your back foot off the floor. As you lift the back leg straight, hinge forwards through your hips so as to lower your trunk, but do not take your shoulders any lower than hip height. Maintain the balance for the exhalation then breathe in and repeat the lunge by lowering your back foot to the floor again. Repeat 8–12 times on each leg.

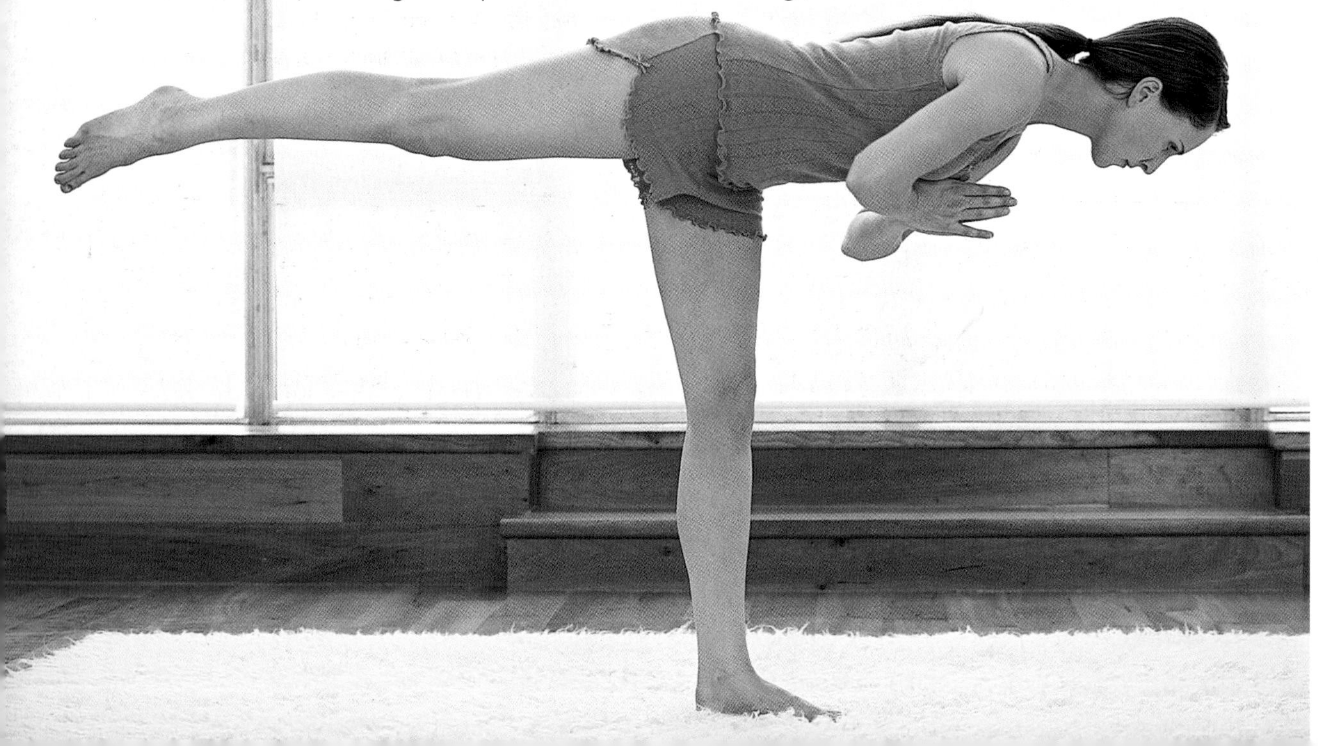

jackknife

This technique strengthens the spine, legs and abdomen with movement.

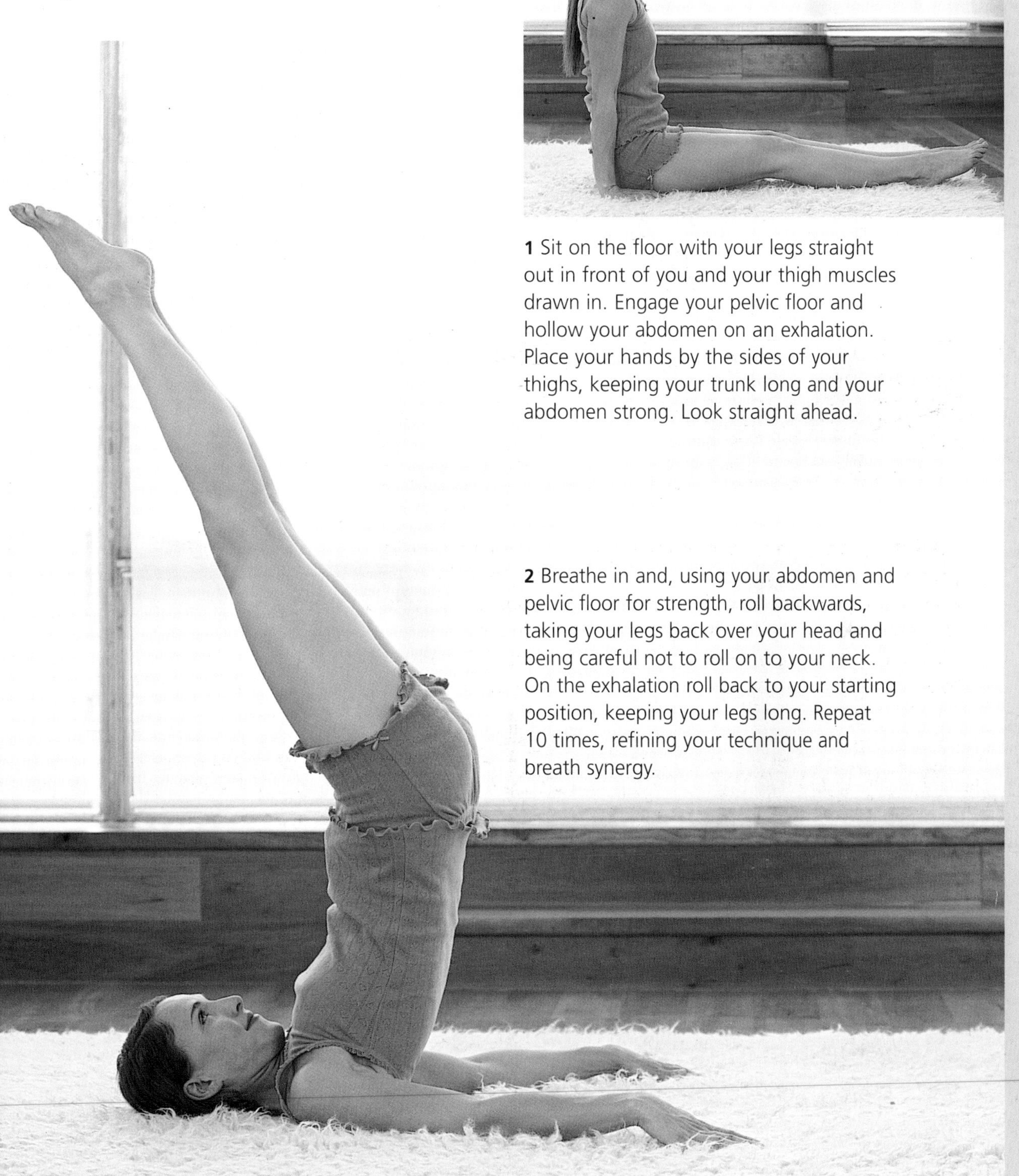

1 Sit on the floor with your legs straight out in front of you and your thigh muscles drawn in. Engage your pelvic floor and hollow your abdomen on an exhalation. Place your hands by the sides of your thighs, keeping your trunk long and your abdomen strong. Look straight ahead.

2 Breathe in and, using your abdomen and pelvic floor for strength, roll backwards, taking your legs back over your head and being careful not to roll on to your neck. On the exhalation roll back to your starting position, keeping your legs long. Repeat 10 times, refining your technique and breath synergy.

arm openers

Use this movement to open the upper body and stretch the chest, but do not perform if you have a disc-related injury.

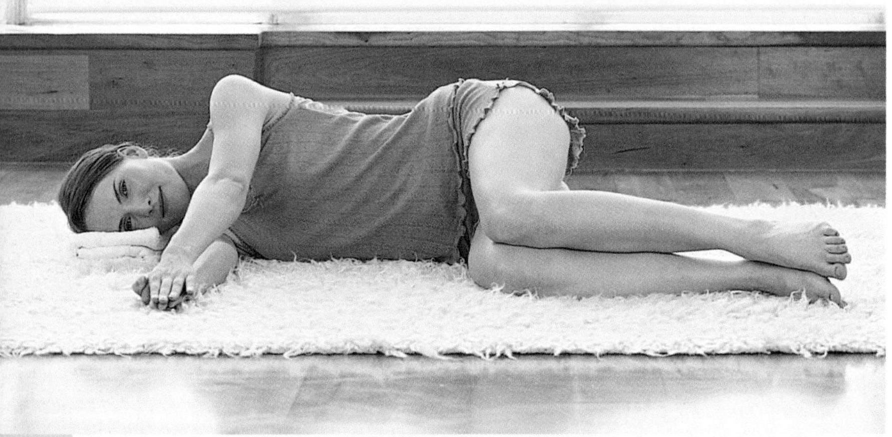

1 Lie on one side with your head on a pillow or rolled-up towel and your knees curled up in front of you at a right angle to your body, your knees and ankles together. Your back should be in a straight line, but keeping its natural curve. Extend your arms in front of you at shoulder height with your palms together.

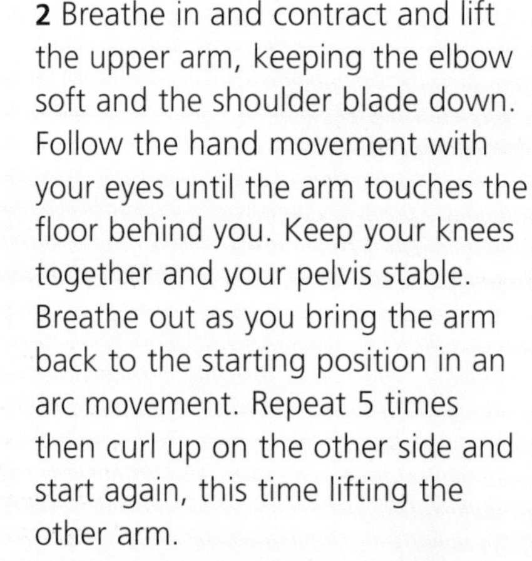

2 Breathe in and contract and lift the upper arm, keeping the elbow soft and the shoulder blade down. Follow the hand movement with your eyes until the arm touches the floor behind you. Keep your knees together and your pelvis stable. Breathe out as you bring the arm back to the starting position in an arc movement. Repeat 5 times then curl up on the other side and start again, this time lifting the other arm.

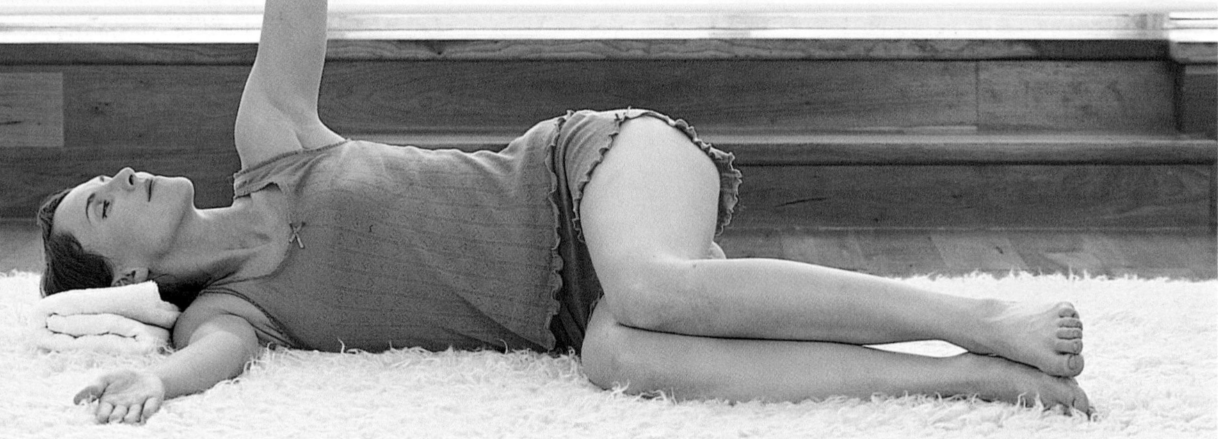

one-leg stretch

This stretch is great for core strength as well as toning the legs. It focuses the breath and improves coordination.

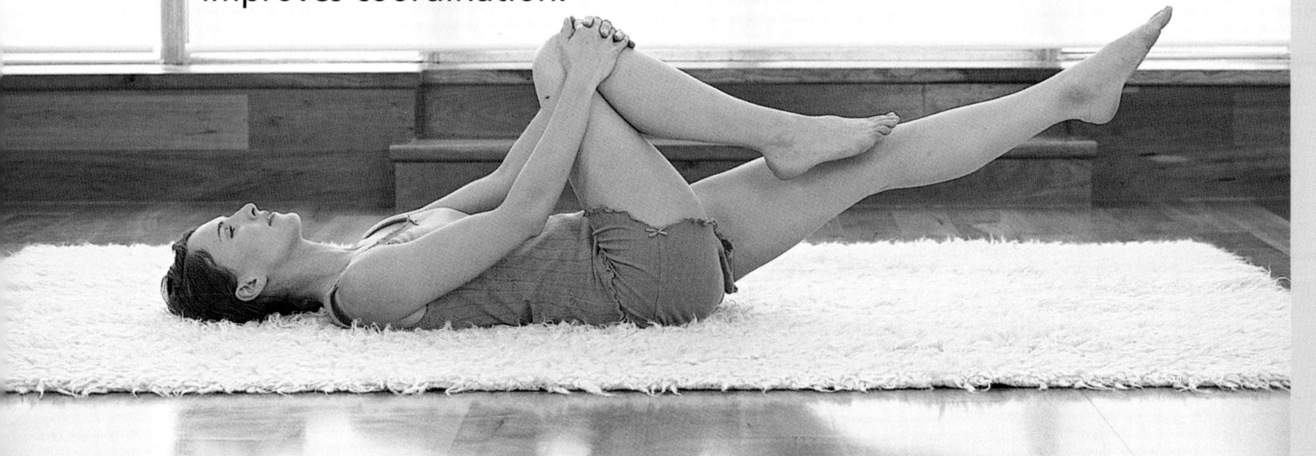

1 Lie on your back on the floor. Bring your right knee in towards your chest and gently hold the shin with both hands while extending your left leg away from the pelvis, slightly raised off the floor. Ensure that your spine is in a neutral position – neither rounded nor arched into the floor.

2 Inhale. As you exhale cycle your legs to change their position so that you bring the left knee in towards your chest. Ensure your spine does not move by hollowing your abdominal muscles. Repeat 15 times then rest with both knees drawn into your chest.

side kick kneeling

This is a great strengthening movement for the shoulders, abdomen, waist and spine while also toning the legs.

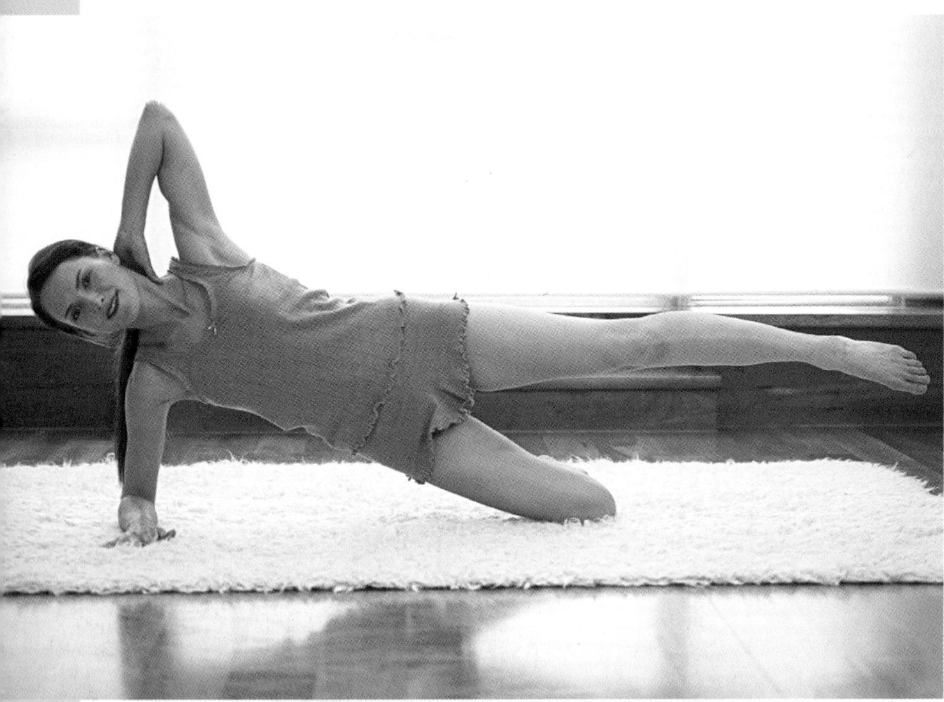

1 Lie on one side with the elbow on that side resting on the floor directly beneath the shoulder and the leg closest to the floor bent behind you with your knees, hips and shoulders all in a line. Inhale. As you exhale draw your abdominals in towards your spine and lift your pelvis off the floor. Stretch out the uppermost leg long and draw the thigh muscle into the thigh bone to engage the thigh. Inhale and extend the uppermost arm upwards above your shoulder then place the hand behind your head.

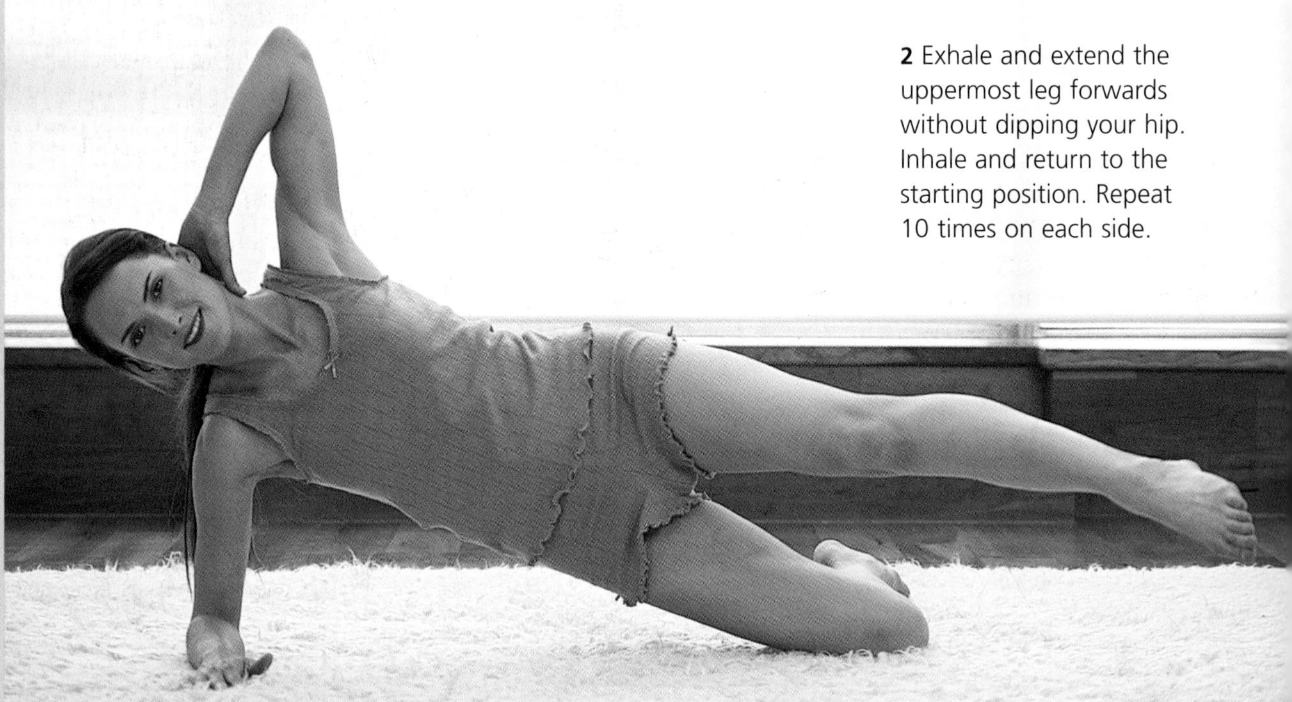

2 Exhale and extend the uppermost leg forwards without dipping your hip. Inhale and return to the starting position. Repeat 10 times on each side.

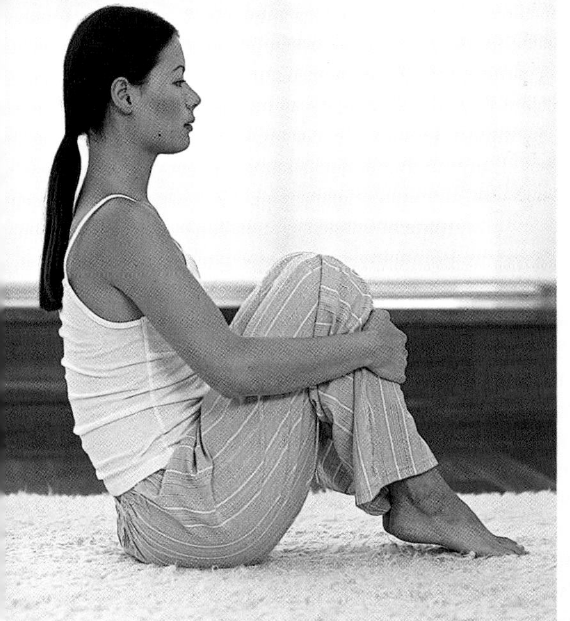

the roll

The rolling movement strengthens the abdominals and spine against the effects of gravity and momentum.

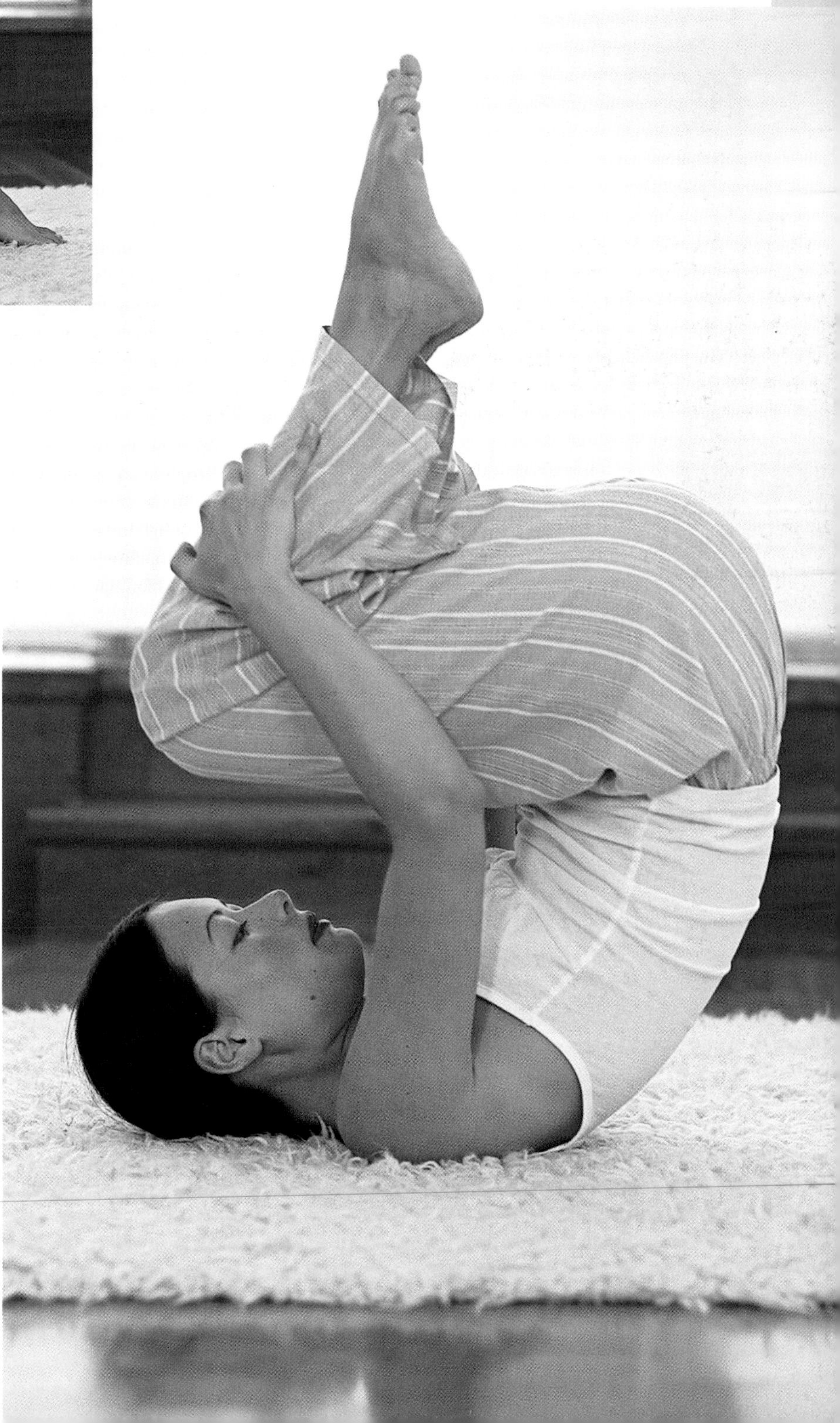

1 Sit on the floor with your knees bent. Maintain a long spine and abdomen. Place your hands on your shins and gently lift your trunk up and out of the pelvis while pulling your abdominals in towards your spine.

2 Breathe in and open your rib cage to allow your lungs to fully inflate. Rock back on to your spine – not your neck – using your arms to push off the floor if necessary. Breathe out and lift your trunk, rolling back to the starting position with a long spine and abdomen. Try not to let your abdominal muscles dome (round out) but keep them taut to stabilize the spine. Repeat 8–12 times, following the correct breathing pattern.

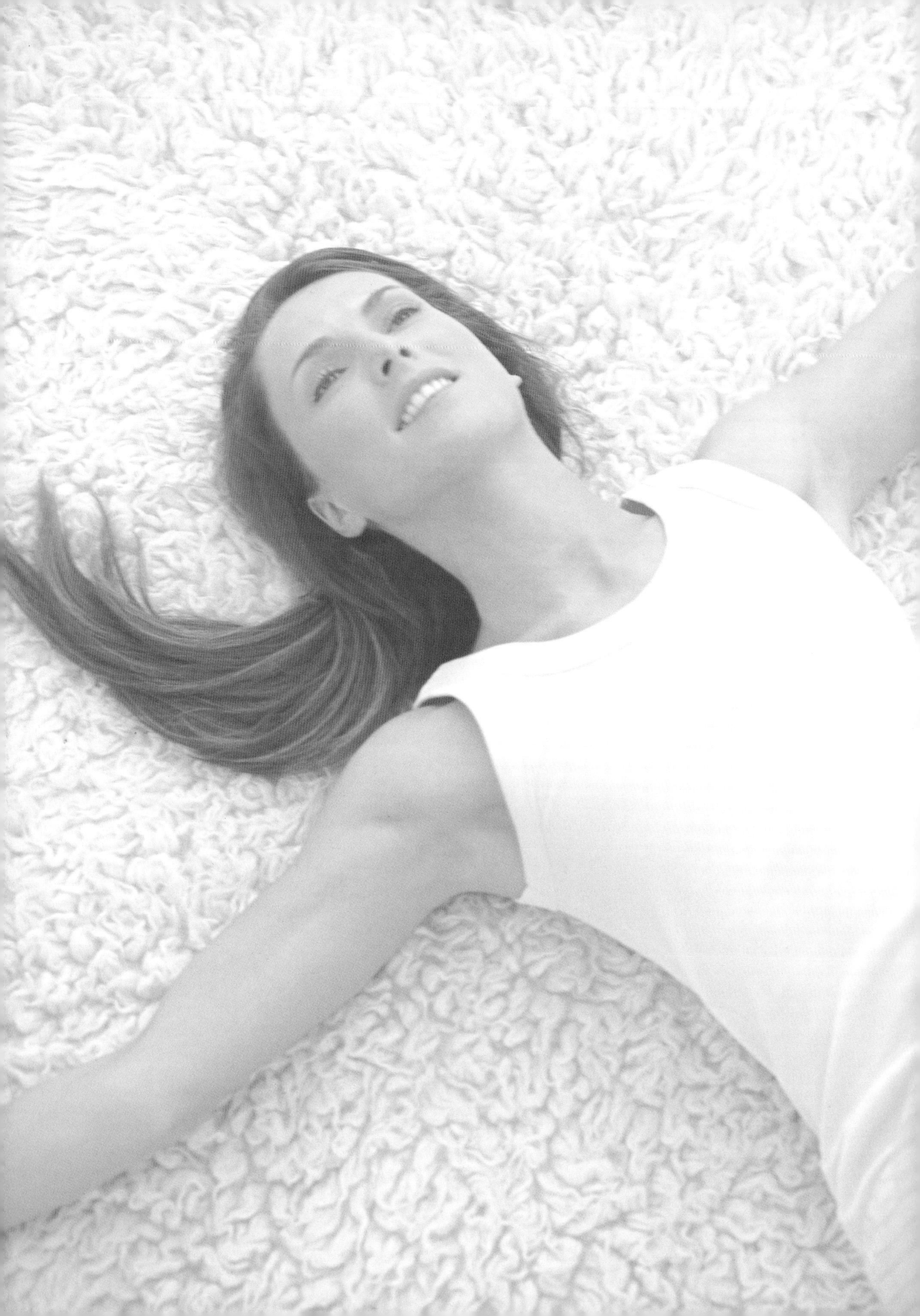

abdominal activators

abdominal activators

The body's trunk is called the 'core' and it is the core that is responsible for holding the body upright in a good posture and from where all movement originates. If your core is out of balance through negative movement patterns then the origin of any movement is also out of alignment. It is therefore important to maintain and service all the muscles in this area in order to prevent tension, stiffness and sagging of the abdominal muscles (known as abs).

Importance of strong abs

Abdominal muscles provide support and protection for your internal organs and help with your breathing, especially exhaling. They also work in conjunction with your back muscles to allow bending and twisting movements. Weak abdominals are usually the cause of back pain or back conditions. This occurs when the transversus abdominis (the lower abdominal muscle, which runs horizontally from one side of the lumbar spine around to the other like a corset) and pelvic floor muscles have not been exercised correctly in synergy with the multifidus (a deep lumbar muscle with a key stabilizing function). Together, these deep stabilizing muscles of your pelvis and spine should act as a corset to your core; if they are weak they cannot protect your spine from unbalanced bone loading – and the result is possible back pain and abdominal sagging.

'The abs exercises will help to firm loose muscles, making you feel taller and more confident'

Your pelvic floor muscles

It is important to practise the 'Pelvic floor elevator' technique described on page 91, because engaging your pelvic floor muscles will help you to tone your abdominals more effectively than just using the abdomen alone. The pelvic floor consists of three main sections – the urogenitals (the front section), the perineum (the middle) and the anus (the back). While performing all of the abdominal exercises featured in this chapter it is the action of gently zipping up the first two pelvic floor sections as you exhale that will give you inner core strength. The result will be flatter abdominal muscles and stronger pelvic floor muscles.

The workout

The exercises in this chapter are very modern and steer clear of the old-school-style abdominal crunches. They are designed to give you maximum output in the 10 minutes available. Good posture is about much more than just standing up straight. These exercises will help to firm loose muscles, making you feel taller and more confident.

NOTE If you have a back condition the movements will help you strengthen the muscles necessary to overcome your condition but you must take care to listen to your body so as not to cause an injury.

BENEFITS OF STRONG ABDOMINALS

- Increased strength and muscular endurance
- Good core stability
- Healthy back
- Improved flexibility
- Toned waist and abdomen

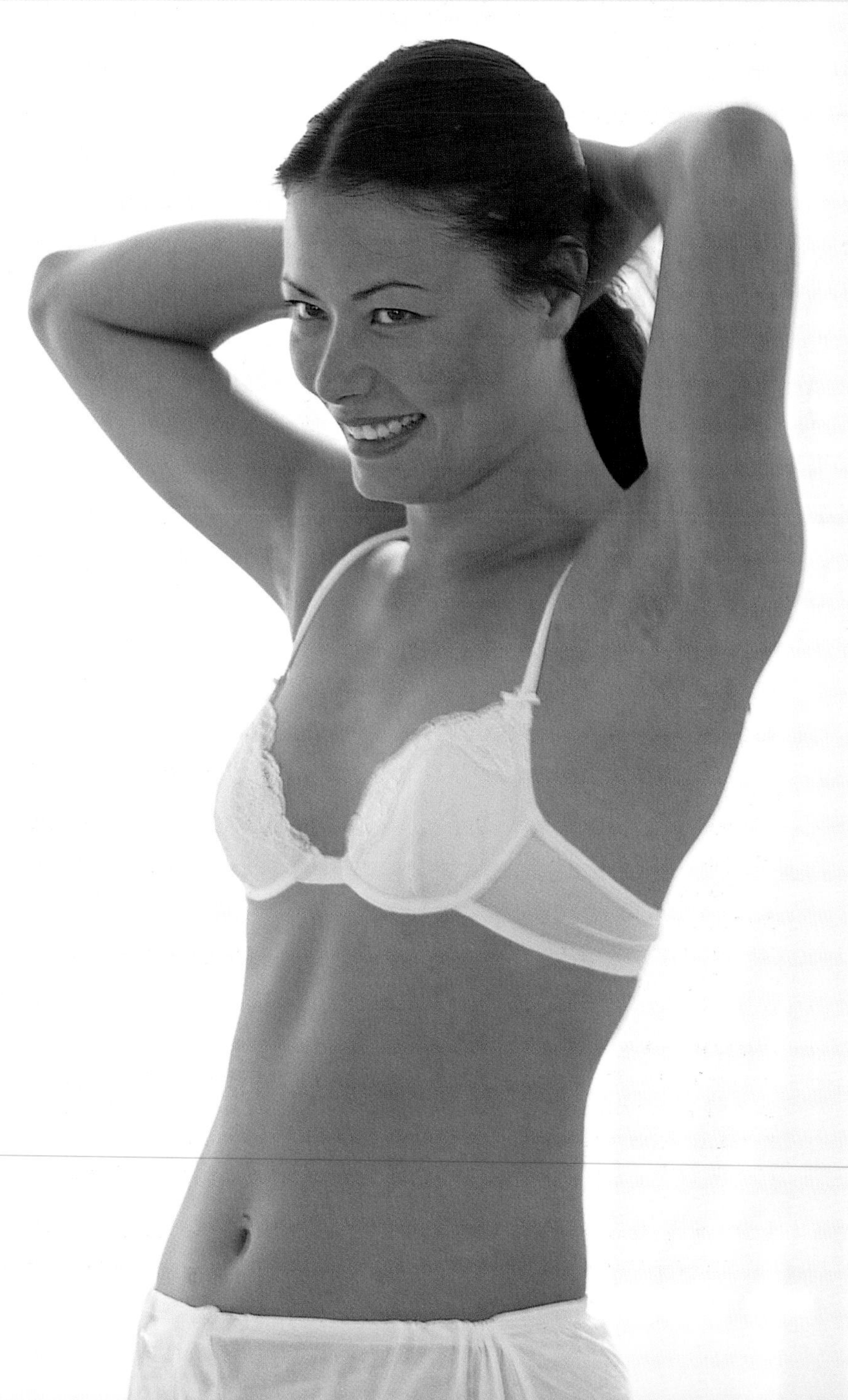

supported V-sit

This abdomen and spine strengthener is the easier version of the exercise opposite as you use your hands for support.

1 Sit on the floor with your knees bent and your feet together, a comfortable distance away from your buttocks. (Your back forms one edge of a 'V' shape and your thighs the other, which explains the name of the exercise.) Inhale. As you exhale draw your abdomen inwards and relax your shoulders away from your ears. Ensure your back is long and strong, not rounded. Put your right hand on your left wrist and grip behind your thighs. Inhale. As you exhale lengthen your spine, lift your feet off the floor and hold for 3–5 cycles of slow breathing.

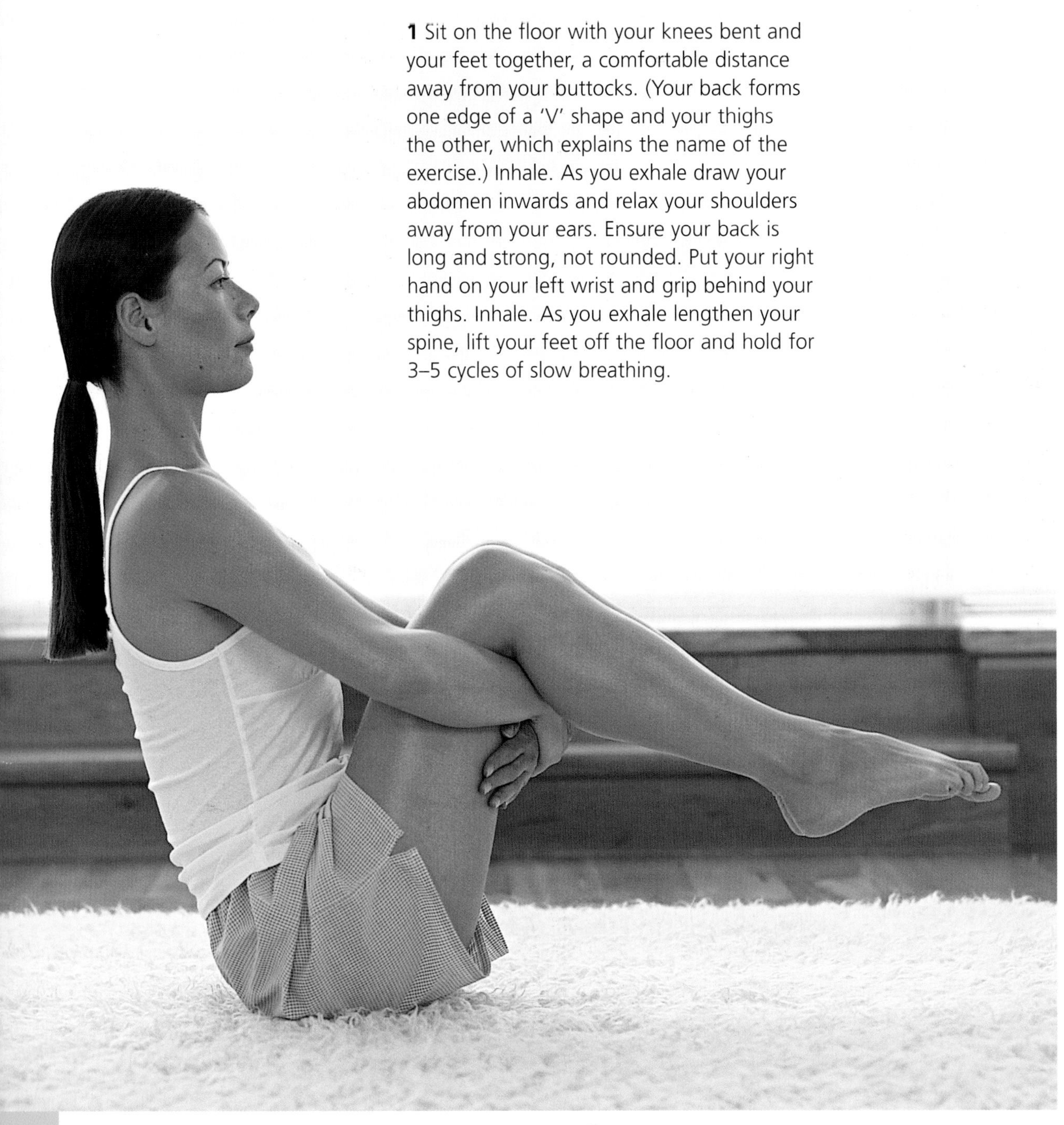

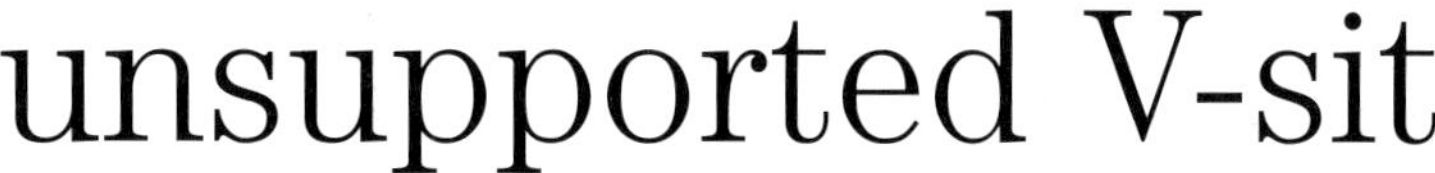

unsupported V-sit

Strengthen your lower back and lower abdominal muscle (transversus abdominis) with this challenging exercise.

1 Sit on the floor with your knees bent and your feet together, a comfortable distance away from your buttocks. Inhale. As you exhale draw your abdomen inwards and relax your shoulders away from your ears. Your back should be long and strong, not rounded. Inhale. As you exhale stretch out your arms in line with your shoulders. Inhale. As you exhale lift both feet off the floor with your knees almost straight. Hold for 3–5 slow cycles of breathing.

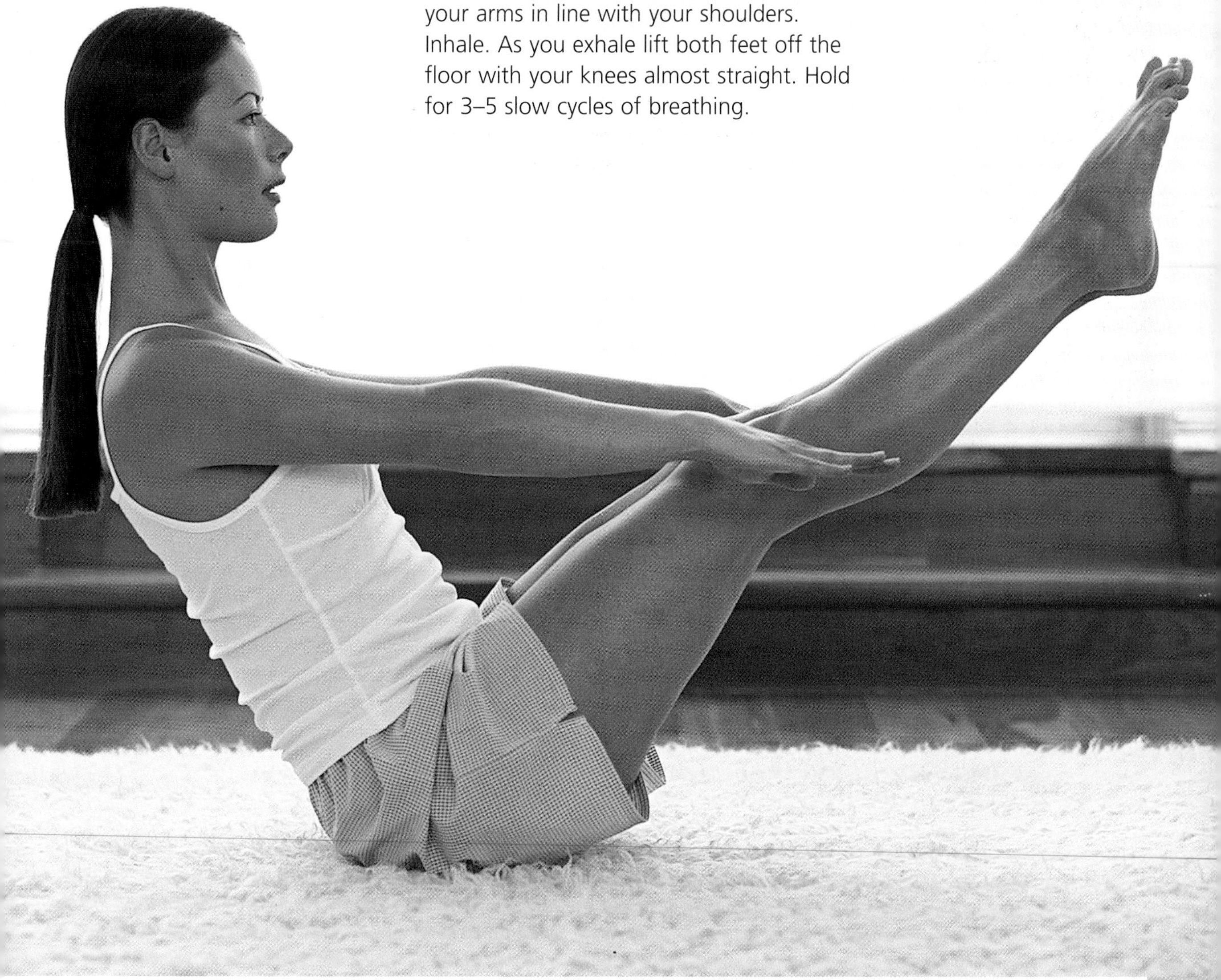

crunches

Crunches help strengthen your abdomen and spine – even more so if you rest your feet on a sofa or chair.

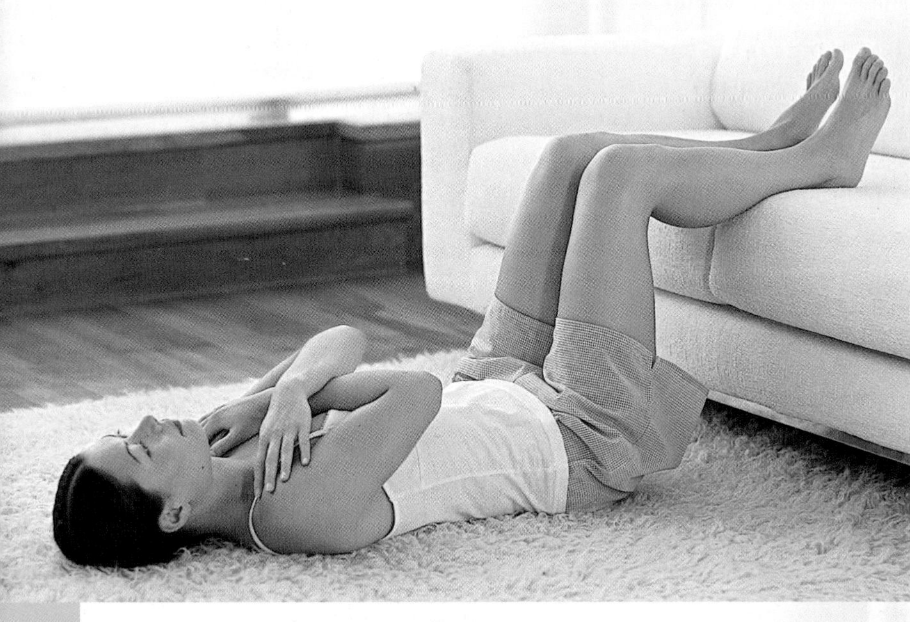

1 Lie on your back on the floor and place your lower legs on the edge of a low bed, sofa or chair. (A Swiss ball is good if you have one as the movement of the ball makes the exercise more challenging and will help strengthen your core stability.) Inhale and cross your arms over your chest, placing your hands flat on your opposite shoulders.

2 Exhale while raising your trunk. Inhale as you release down, then exhale and lift back up. Repeat 20 times, following the correct breathing pattern.

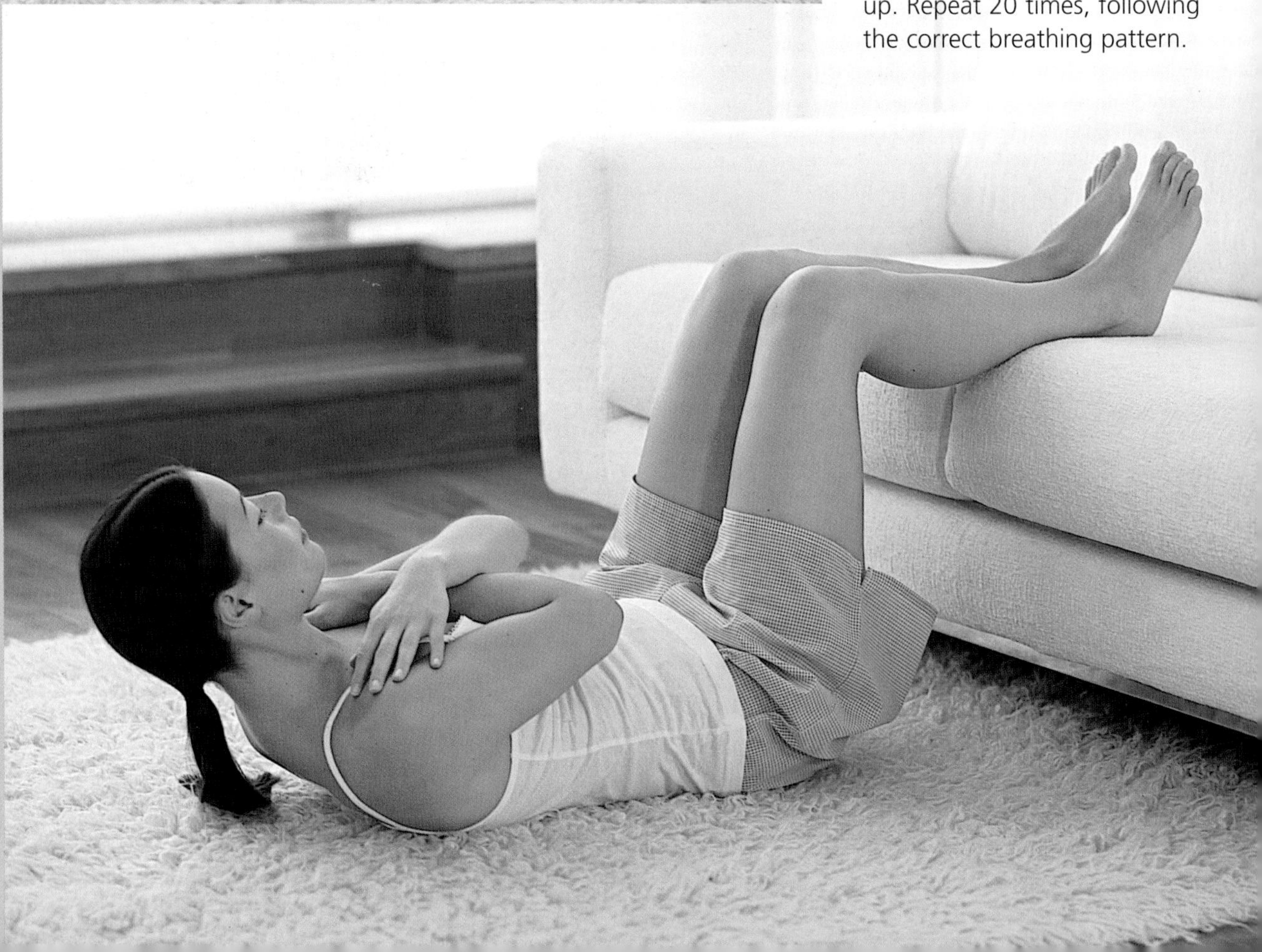

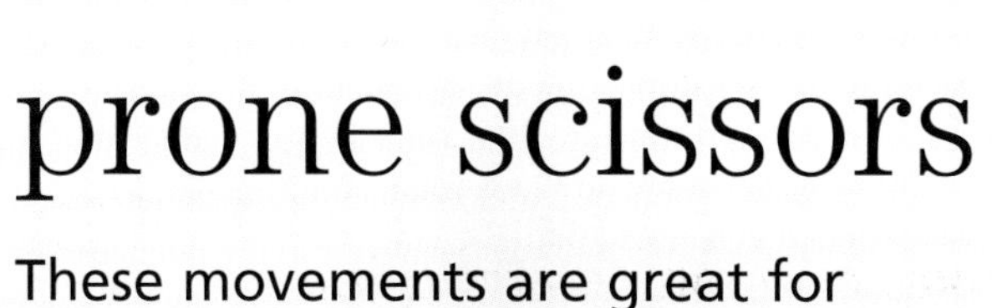

prone scissors

These movements are great for improving circulation in the legs while firming your abdomen.

1 Lie on your back with both legs straight in the air, shoulder width apart, and your arms stretched out to your sides. Engage your abdomen and draw your thigh muscles into your thigh bones.

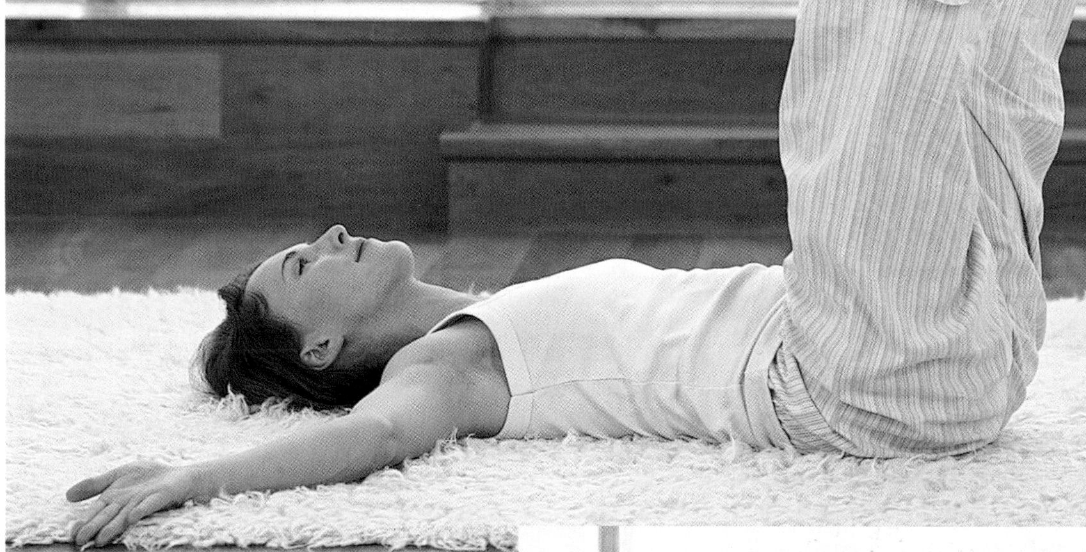

2 Inhale and criss-cross your legs over one another, like scissors, then exhale and bring them back to the starting position. Repeat the criss-crossing of your legs for 15 separate repetitions, following the correct breathing pattern.

waist twist

These gentle twists tone the waist muscles and spine.

1 Lie on your back with your legs off the floor, your knees bent at right angles, and your arms stretched out on the floor beyond your head.

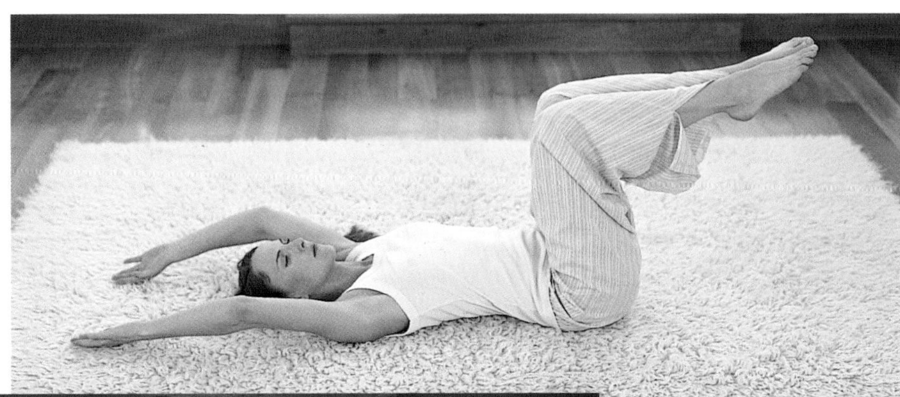

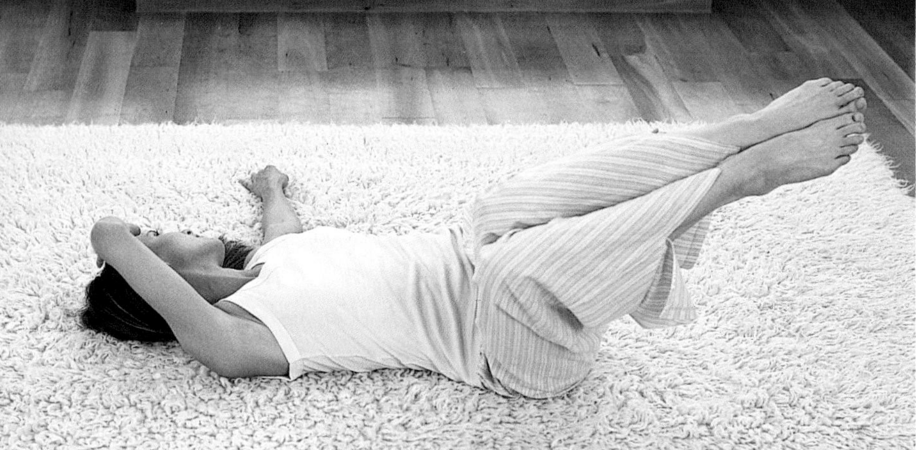

2 Inhale. As you exhale take your legs over to the right and your arms to the left but do not let either rest on the floor. Inhale as you bring your legs and arms back to the centre.

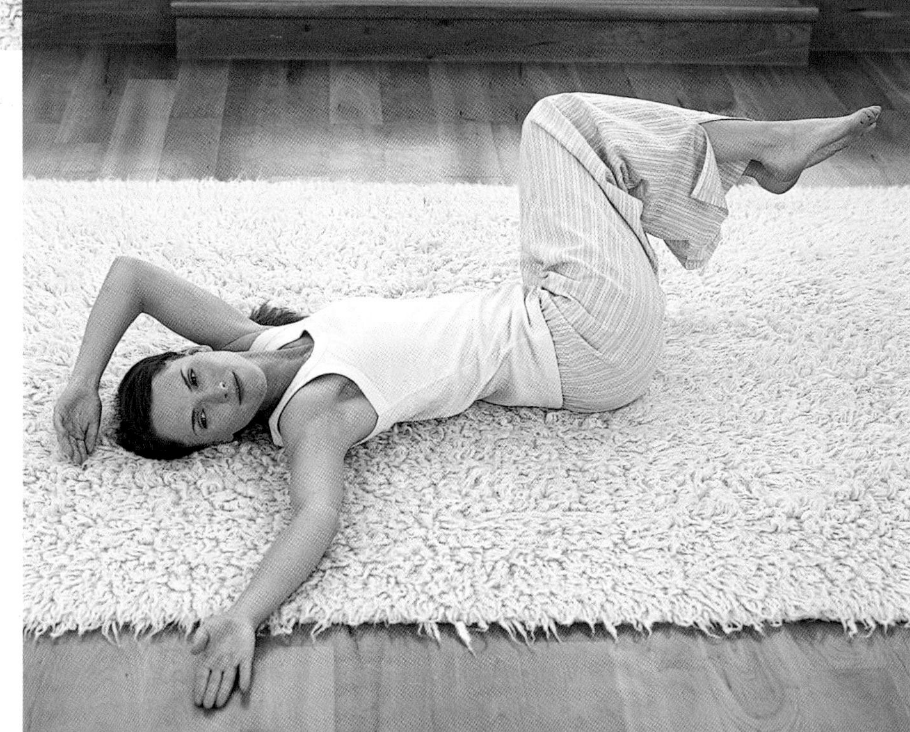

3 Exhale and repeat the movement, this time taking your legs over to the left and your arms to the right. Repeat 10 times, following the correct breathing pattern.

roll-downs

This exercise uses gravity to help you establish a deep abdominal strength.

1 Lie on your back on the floor with your knees drawn towards your chest and your arms down by your sides, palms facing down.

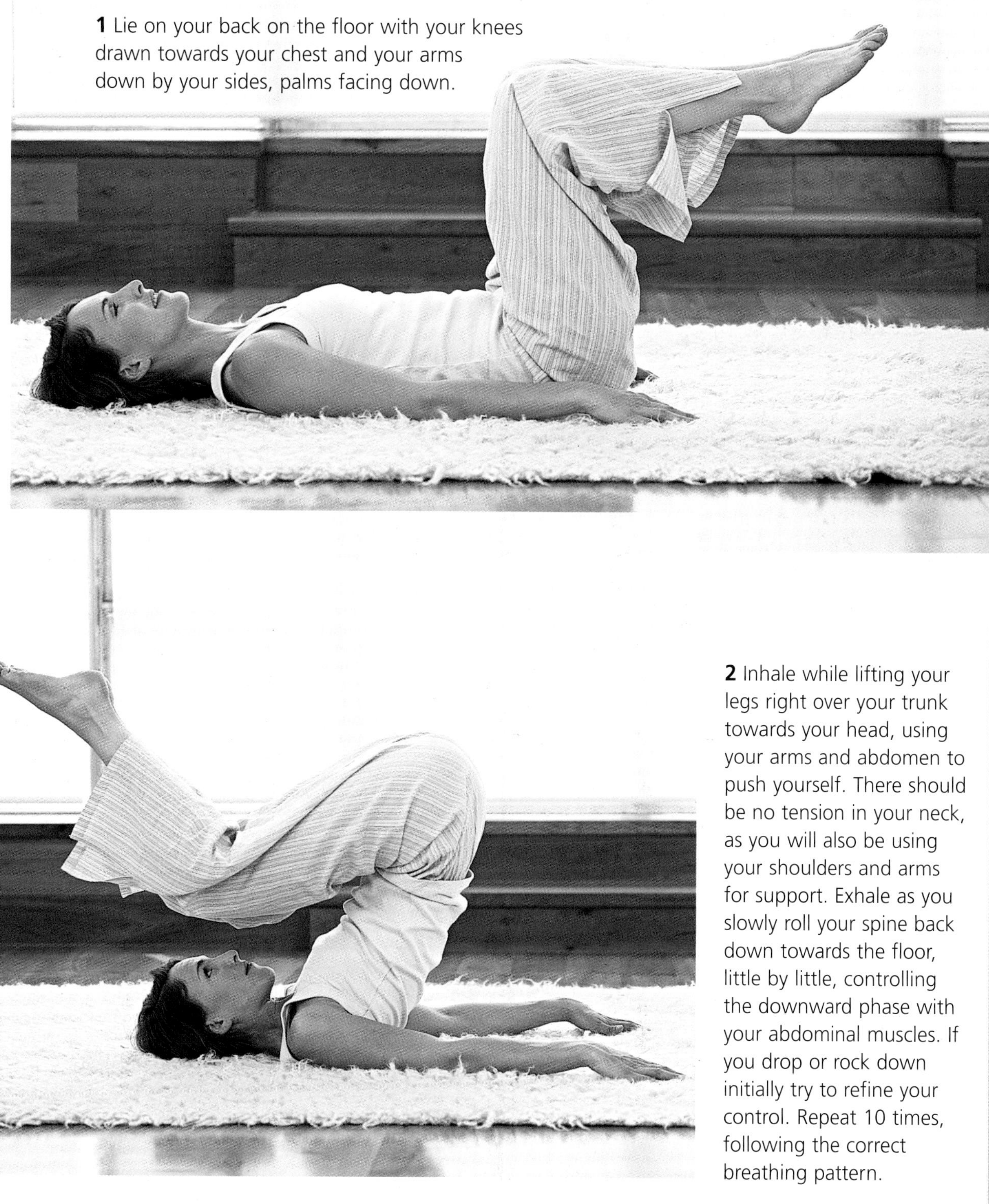

2 Inhale while lifting your legs right over your trunk towards your head, using your arms and abdomen to push yourself. There should be no tension in your neck, as you will also be using your shoulders and arms for support. Exhale as you slowly roll your spine back down towards the floor, little by little, controlling the downward phase with your abdominal muscles. If you drop or rock down initially try to refine your control. Repeat 10 times, following the correct breathing pattern.

index

acknowledgements

Executive Editor Jane McIntosh
Managing Editor Clare Churly
Executive Art Editor Joanna MacGregor
Designer Maggie Town, one2six creative
Photographer Russell Sadur
Production Controller Nigel Reed
Models Jackie Chan and Sally Lovegrove